COMMUNITY PHARMACY PRACTICE

COMMUNITY PHARMACY PRACTICE

Dr. Ramesh Adepu
M.Pharm, Ph.D
Professor, Department of Pharmacy Practice,
JSS College of Pharmacy, SS Nagar,
Mysore -15, India.

PharmaMed Press
An imprint of Pharma Book Syndicate
A unit of BSP Books Pvt. Ltd.
4-4-309/316, Giriraj Lane,
Sultan Bazar, Hyderabad - 500 095.

Community Pharmacy Practice by *Adepu Ramesh*

Published by

PharmaMed Press
An imprint of Pharma Book Syndicate
A unit of BSP Books Pvt. Ltd.
4-4-309/316, Giriraj Lane, Sultan Bazar, Hyderabad - 500 095.
Phone: 040-23445605, 23445688; Fax: 91+40-23445611
E-mail: info@pharmamedpress.com

ISBN: 978-93-85433-90-0 (HB)

Dedicated to the Lotus Feet of My Spiritual Master

Sri Baba Anwarananda Maharaj

and

Poojya Mathrusri

PHARMACY COUNCIL OF INDIA

(Constituted under the Pharmacy Act. 1948)

Prof. B. Suresh, **M.Pharm, Ph.D., D.sc.**
President

Combined Council's Building
Kotla Road, Alwan-E-Ghalib Marg
P.B. No. 7020, New Delhi-110 002
Gram: Farmcouncil
Tel: 011 23239184, 23231348
Fax: 011 23239184

Vice-Chancellor, JSS Univerisity
JSS Medical Institutions Campus
S.S. Nagar, Mysore 570 015
Tel: 0821 2548391
Fax: 0821 2548394
Sureshbhojraj@hotmail.com
Sureshjssuni@hotmail.com
www.jssuni.edu.in

FOREWORD

Community Pharmacy Practice is an amalgam of business and patient care practice. The business component of community Pharmacy includes trade related activities such as procurement, inventory management, and accounting. Patient care activities include review of prescriptions, dispensing, counseling, health screening, and drug therapy management. Thus community pharmacy practice is a science and an art. In order to understand the concept and develop the necessary skills, a separate textbook on community pharmacy practice is the need of hour.

The textbook of community pharmacy practice is divided into nineteen chapters covering the scope of the community pharmacy practice, pharmaceutical care, patient counseling activity, patient information leaflets, health screening services, community pharmacy management, inventory control management, role of community pharmacist in health promotion, contraception, immunization and management of minor ailments, Pharmacovigilance in community pharmacy and research in community pharmacy. The content covered in the textbook will meet the academic needs of students pursuing diploma, Pharm D and M. Pharm in Pharmacy Practice studying community pharmacy practice as a separate subject.

The Author has put good amount of time and efforts in writing this textbook to give the best information and justification to the title of the book. I wish him the best and good luck for future endeavors.

Dr. B. Suresh
President
Pharmacy Council of India
& Vice Chancellor, JSS University, Mysore.

PREFACE

In India, community pharmacy always referred as retail pharmacy where the primary focus is trade. Although the concept of pharmacy practice is well defined and appreciated and practiced in western part of the world since 90's, while in India, the pharmacy practice is still an unaware concept. Reasons for this situation are plenty. One among them is, from the beginning of the pharmacy education, major focus was given to industry oriented subjects. Patient focused concept was realized with introduction of clinical pharmacy education in India since 1996. Unfortunately lack of trained staff, non availability of the textbooks to meet the academic needs of students studying pharmacy practice was a big challenge. To overcome this challenge, a sincere effort was made to bring out a textbook on community pharmacy practice.

The textbook of community pharmacy practice contains nineteen chapters. The content in the book is primarily focused to cover the syllabus of Community Pharmacy Practice subject of Pharm D. Apart from that additional chapters such as Pharmacovigilance in community pharmacies, research in community pharmacy practice was given to support the learning of post graduate students in Community Pharmacy Practice and to design research works in the area of community pharmacy. All chapters are given with learning objectives, text on the concept, key points, case studies where necessary to make the student to understand the concept and skills necessary for practice and suggested further reading to assist the students to maximize their learning.

As a student, as a teacher-practitioner the difficulty I faced to understand the concept of community pharmacy practice, the research components in community pharmacy has motivated me to write a textbook on Community Pharmacy Practice. I have taken almost two years to complete this book. My heart felt thanks to my beloved spiritual master Sri Baba Anwarananda Maharaj for motivating me to pursue my higher studies. My sincere thanks to my teacher, my mentor and guide Dr. B.G.Nagavi who was inspirational for me to choose my Ph.D research work in Community Pharmacy Practice area and made me to realize the academic needs in the community pharmacy practice. My thanks to my best friend, teacher and colleague Dr. G. Parthasarathi, who always motivated me to a make mark in the community pharmacy practice in India and giving me an opportunity to write a chapter in his text book of Clinical Pharmacy Practice, which I have taken as model in designing my text book. My sincere thanks to my best friend and the practicing community pharmacist Mr. Raj Vaidya, who reviewed few chapters and gave critical comments to strengthen the content in the chapters. My deepest thanks also go to my department colleagues and well wishers who always supported me in writing this book. My hearty thanks to BS Publications, who came forward to publish this textbook.

Last but not the least my family members especially my wife Swaroopa Rani, and children Pawan and Vivek who sacrificed many important occasions while I was on this task.

I have made my sincere efforts to give the best possible information to justify the title of the chapter and overall as textbook. I whole heartedly welcome any critical comments from my colleagues and well wishers regarding the deficiencies in the chapter which I should have covered etc., or any other new points. I will certainly try to overcome all those in my next edition and also probably I will also add more new and current concepts in the area of community pharmacy practice.

Ramesh Adepu

CONTENTS

Chapter 18
RESEARCH IN COMMUNITY PHARMACY PRACTICE

CHAPTER 19
CODE OF ETHICS FOR COMMUNITY PHARMACISTS

CHAPTER 1

COMMUNITY PHARMACY PRACTICE – AN INTRODUCTION

LEARNING OBJECTIVES

- Define community pharmacy and community pharmacist
- Know the scope of community pharmacy practice
- Understand the professional roles of community pharmacists

INTRODUCTION

From ancient days, medicines are being used to treat various ailments. Medicines are prepared using plant, animal and mineral sources. The Apothecaries, who were the trained individuals, compounded and dispensed the medicines against the prescriptions given by the physicians. Availability of modern prepackaged medicines has slowly eliminated the compounding activities of the pharmacists. Thus the pharmacists are confined to dispensing activity both in hospital and community setting. However over the years, worldwide pharmacists have gained a special recognition due to their patient focused services.

Definition

Community Pharmacy is defined as a place where the medicines are stocked and dispensed to the patients on a valid prescription and where legally permitted without a prescription and also offer various professional services that improves the health of the patient.

Community pharmacists are the health care professionals easily accessible to the public and supply medicines in accordance with a prescription or sell them without a prescription when legally permitted. In addition to ensuring an accurate supply of appropriate medicines and health care products, their professional activities include patient counseling, dissemination of unbiased drug information, providing clinical pharmacy services, and health promotion.

World Health Organisation (W.H.O) defines ***Community Pharmacist*** as legally qualified, trained health care professional who act as a vital link between the patient and the prescriber. The pharmacist ensures the correct supply of medicines and provides medication usage information both to patients and prescribers and helps in minimizing the drug related problems through clinical pharmacy services.

SCOPE

An occupation possessing special attributes characterized by power, knowledge, and autonomy is called as a profession. An individual possessing knowledge and concerned with providing services to the client, patient or to the community is called as professional. Among health care professions, medical profession from the beginning dominated the other health related occupations, by virtue of subordination, limitation, and exclusion. Nursing is an example of subordination in medicine since nurses directly work under the doctors. Dentistry and Pharmacy are examples of limitation, because dentistry is limited to a part of the body, where as pharmacy limits to a therapeutic technique. Alternate practice of medicine such as Chiropody, and Osteopathy are the examples of exclusion, since they do not have any official recognition. Doctor's dominance is preserved by their capacity to determine the overall parameters of the division of labor. But in recent times, other branches such as physiotherapy, which has achieved some autonomy in the health care system, posing challenges to the dominance of doctors.

PHARMACY AS A PROFESSION

There is a broad agreement that pharmacy is an underdeveloped profession due to limitation by the authority of the doctor who delegates the pharmacist with the medical division of labor. The traditional activities of the pharmacists include preparation of various dosage forms, maintaining the stability and strength, ensuring that the drug is extracted and prepared in such a way to maximize its therapeutic properties under safe storage practices. With the technical advancement in pharmaceutical industry, and bulk production of pharmaceutical formulations, dispensing of prescriptions has become the major job function of the pharmacists. During early days, pharmacists were underutilized despite pharmacists' authority on drugs and were not included in the health care team. Automation of tablet counting and computerization of dispensing, and trader approaches of community pharmacists, have become hurdles in recognition of community pharmacist as a health care professional.

The Nuffield inquiry report in 1986 established the need for community pharmacists' to improve their professional knowledge, and skills to interpret the therapeutic regimens for drug related issues and counsel the patients to get recognition from the medical professionals. Researchers have identified the need of reprofessionalisation among the pharmacists through acquiring the knowledge of clinical skills such as direct involvement in drug therapy decisions through monitoring the patient case notes, laboratory investigation details, adverse drug reactions and counseling of patients about the optimal use of medications and providing unbiased information on drugs.

The development of clinical pharmacy in 80's has provided some individualization to the pharmacy profession. During the early days though the doctors were antagonistic to the pharmacists' therapeutic intervention activities later realized the importance of therapeutic advisory roles of the clinical pharmacists.

In 1973, Linn and Davis focused on the importance of developing new professional roles for the community pharmacists in order to improve their self worth and job satisfaction. Attempts were made in the direction to improve professionalization in community pharmacies through patient counseling and pharmacist role in maximizing the patient medication adherence.

INTERNATIONAL SCENARIO OF COMMUNITY PHARMACY PRACTICE

Globally pharmacy profession has undergone significant changes in the recent decades. It has shifted the focus from the product to the patient. The role of the pharmacist has changed from that of a commander and supplier of pharmaceutical products to that of a provider of services and information and ultimately as a provider of patient care through pharmaceutical care services.

Linn and Davis stressed upon the importance of developing new roles for community pharmacists in order to meet the professional challenges and gain recognition as a health care professional. As a result, community pharmacists in developed countries like Australia, U.S, and U.K have accepted the new professional responsibilities apart from dispensing. The new roles of the community pharmacists include medication record review, medication usage counseling, unbiased drug information, home medication review, health screening services, and education on smoking cessation and family planning.

In the USA, practicing pharmacists have developed a smoking cessation program for the patients in cooperation with National Cancer Institute. They have also engaged in screening and counseling of Diabetes and Hypertension patients, detection, and prevention of Cancer, education on family planning and sexually transmitted diseases.

In U.K, pharmacists are engaged in health education programs to the public about safe use of medicines, dental health, prevention of coronary diseases and patient compliance with the help of posters, leaflets, badges, and audiovisual displays as information sources. Other services they offered to the public were screening of blood pressure and cholesterol and providing necessary information to the patients. These services are showing a positive impact on the patient's health.

In Australia, community pharmacists are offering wide range of activities, such as home medication reviews, population screening and testing for hypertension, glaucoma, and diabetis apart from providing necessary patient counseling on drugs and diseases.

INDIAN SCENARIO OF COMMUNITY PHARMACY PRACTICE

In India, community pharmacy is often referred as "Medical & General Store". As per the legal requirement to open a pharmacy, a qualified person or "Registered Pharmacist" is required under section 42 of Drugs & Cosmetic Act and all dispensing activities are expected to be carried out in presence of the pharmacist. In India, minimum qualification for registration as "pharmacist" is Diploma in Pharmacy (D.Pharm) where as in majority of developed countries, the minimum qualification required for registration is B.Pharm or Pharm D. A strict legal enforcement is practiced to dispense the medications only by the pharmacist. Unfortunately in India, pharmacists are not seen physically in majority of community pharmacies. In a study conducted in Mysore by R Adepu *et al.*, about 68% of pharmacies in Mysore city did not have the physical presence of the pharmacist while dispensing the medicines. Major activity that happens in the pharmacies is prescription filling only. Often this prescription filling is done by the non qualified persons who basically treat the pharmacy profession as trade.

ROLES AND RESPONSIBILITIES OF COMMUNITY PHARMACIST

The consultative group of the World Health Organization listed the following responsibilities as the professional responsibilities of the community pharmacists. The International Pharmaceutical Federation also confirms the same.

- Processing of the prescriptions
- Dispensing
- Patient counseling
- Drug information services
- Health promotion
- Health screening services
- Responding to symptoms of minor ailments
- Consultation to General Practitioners

Processing of the Prescriptions

Pharmacists are expected to review and check the prescriptions for the legality, appropriateness and potential drug related problems in the prescription. Upon satisfaction with the content of the prescription, the pharmacist will dispense the prescribed medicines.

Dispensing

The meaning of "dispensing" according to Oxford dictionary is to make up and give out the medicines on a prescription. In the early days as the pharmacists were engaged in compounding activity, the prescribed medicines were appropriately compounded and dispensed to the patient. Currently, prepackaged medicines as various pharmaceutical dosage forms are available in the market, thus the compounding and dispensing activity has become obsolete. Thus the pharmacist should label each item prescribed in the prescription with the name of the patient, age, gender, name of the drug, instructions for proper use of the drug, name of the prescriber and the seal of the pharmacy.

Patient Counseling

Majority of the patients may not have proper ideas about the correct usage of their medicines. Due to their busy schedules and over patient load, often prescribers may give very brief information about the medicines. Thus it is an opportunity for the pharmacists to step into the counseling role.

Patient counseling is defined as providing the disease related and medication related information in layman language to the patients or patient's representative for appropriate use of prescribed medication and controlling the disease symptoms by practicing an appropriate diet and lifestyle modifications as per the individual requirements.

Many research studies have corroborated the positive influence of counseling in disease management and improved medication adherence behavior and ultimately on improved therapeutic outcomes and health related quality of life.

Drug Information Services

Every year many new molecules are approved by the regulatory authorities and permit the pharmaceutical companies to market them for the labeled indications. However efficacy and the safety profile of these new molecules is often ambiguous. In such situations, prescribers depend on pharmaceutical companies for medication related information. Due to the commercial interests, the information given by the companies in product literature is product favored and biased. To overcome this problem, the pharmacist may take the responsibility to provide unbiased information about the drugs. Drug information is defined as the systematic approach of reviewing various sources of published literature, evaluating the published information and providing the suitable answer to the requester. To provide the information, pharmacist may use various resources such as primary sources (peer reviewed journals e.g., LANCET, BMJ, Annals of Pharmacotherapy etc.), secondary resources (Various databases like IDIS, MicroMedex etc.,) and tertiary resources such as text books and compendia.

Health Promotion

Pharmacists by virtue of their knowledge, skills and the rapport with the public, they will be able to educate the individuals to practice healthy habits and lifestyle practices to prevent diseases. Health promotion activities include smoking cessation programs, family planning, participation in vaccination program and education about deworming and balanced diet.

Health Screening Service

Health screening service is the patient care service that is offered by the pharmacists in community pharmacies. Health screening service plays an important role in early detection of the chronic diseases, and thereby patient can receive early treatment and prevent the complications of the disease. By offering health screening service, community pharmacists can also involve in monitoring and managing the chronic disorders like hypertension, diabetes mellitus, hyperlipdemia, asthma. This will minimize the disease burden on the individual and also on the society. Monitoring refers to observation and in some cases intervention of the disease condition after the diagnosis and treatment, which helps to assess and improve the therapeutic outcomes.

Responding to Symptoms of Minor Ailments

Worldwide pharmacists are known as easily accessible health care professionals to the common man on matters related to the health. When required in case of minor ailments such as common colds, diarrhea, simple body aches, spasms and sprains, pharmacists will be able to give suitable medications to alleviate the symptoms.

Consultation to General Practitioners

Pharmacists by virtue of their professional liaison, they can guide patients to the general practitioners for suitable management of the medical condition. When required pharmacists will provide the drug information to the doctors, supply the emergency drugs to clinics and nursing homes. In Australia, pharmacists in consultation with the general practitioners, participate in home medicine review programs (HMR). HMR is a specialized service offered by accredited community pharmacists. In HMR activity, the HMR pharmacist in consultation with the general practitioners will visit the patients at their residences by taking their appointment. During the house visit, HMR pharmacist review the patient case notes and medications to identify any drug related problems and resolve the same in consultation with the general practitioners and educate the patient appropriately for increased medication adherence and better therapeutic outcomes.

KEY POINTS

- Community Pharmacists are the health care professionals easily accessible to the public and supply the medicines according to the prescriptions and where legally permitted without the prescription for minor ailments as over the counter (OTC) drugs.
- The scope of the community pharmacist has changed from medicine dispenser to pharmaceutical care provider.
- Various professional associations across the world have developed professional standards for their community pharmacists for better patient care services and for professional recognition.
- Important professional roles of the community pharmacists include processing of the prescriptions, dispensing of the medicines, patient counseling, drug information services, health promotion, responding to symptoms of minor ailments and referral of the patients to general practitioners.

SUGGESTED READINGS

1. A. Ramesh, B. G. Nagavi and K. V. Ramanath, Critical review of community Pharmacies (Drug stores) in Mysore city. Indian J Hosp Pharm; 2000 ; May – June : 91 – 93.
2. Bloom MZ (1990). Clinical Pharmacy services improve patient care and reduce costs. *American Pharmacy* NS **30:** 17 - 18.

3. Hepler CD, Strand LM (1990). Opportunities, and responsibilities in pharmaceutical care. *Am J Hosp Pharm.* **47:** 533 - 543.
4. Maddock DH (1990). Potential influential role of the community pharmacists. *Pharm. J* **245:** 233-234.
5. Michael Tatchel, Angela Shepherd (2003). Health care and community pharmacy in Australia. *Pharmacy Review.* **27(3):** AE 2 - AE 4.
6. Mitchell R E, Smart JD, Herring C N (1989). Extended role and the community pharmacist. *Pharm. J* **243:** R 42.
7. Richard K Lewis, Nancy L Lasack, Bruce L Lambert and Sharon E Conner (1997). Patient counseling – a focus on maintenance therapy. *Am J health System Pharm.* **54:** 2084 - 98.
8. The Role of the Pharmacist in the health care system, W.H.O. Consultative group 1993: p. 16-19.
9. Turner P (1984). Pharmacy: An inquiry into contribution to health care. *Bare MED J.* **288:** 810 - 811.
10. USP medication counseling behavior guidelines, USPDI update, 1997: p. 664 – 675.

CHAPTER **2**

PHARMACEUTICAL CARE

LEARNING OBJECTIVES

- Know the definition of "Pharmaceutical Care"
- Understand various types of drug related problems
- Appreciate the steps involved in pharmaceutical care
- Understand and carry out pharmaceutical care activity

INTRODUCTION

Health is defined as physical, mental, and social well being of an individual. Medicines are used to treat various disorders. Medicines if appropriately used will give relief to patients and cause harm to the individual's health if inappropriately used and increases the therapy related expenditures to patients and to the government.

Worldwide pharmacists are offering professional services in community, hospital and clinical setting to meet the patients' pharmaceutical requirements. By virtue of their knowledge in the area of therapeutics and clinical pharmacy, pharmacists are able to identify drug related problems and provide suitable solutions to the patients and as counselors educate the patients about safe usage of their medicines, appropriate diet and life style changes to maximize the therapeutic benefit.

Pharmaceutical public health has been defined as the application of the pharmaceutical knowledge, skills and resources to prevent diseases and prolong the life through promoting, protecting and improving the health of the society in an organized way. Pharmaceutical public health addresses the health related issues at societal level where as pharmaceutical care addresses the health related issues at individual level.

PHARMACEUTICAL CARE

The word "Pharmaceutical Care" was first coined by Mikeal et. al, in 1975 and defined Pharmaceutical care as "the care that a given patient requires and receives which assures safe and rational drug use".

Since 1975, this definition underwent various modifications. In 1990, Duglas C Hepler and Linda M Strand gave a new definition to pharmaceutical care which is globally accepted.

Hepler & Strand defined "Pharmaceutical care as the responsible provision of drug therapy for the purpose of achieving definite outcomes that improves the patient's quality of life". This definition was considered to be more realistic, goal oriented and particularly for chronic diseases such as diabetes, where maintenance of quality of life is an important consideration. In 1998, International Pharmaceutical Federation (FIP) adopted this definition.

The practice of pharmaceutical care is a new concept in contrast to the present practices of the pharmacists. In routine practice, pharmacists dispense the medicines against a prescription. But in pharmaceutical care practice, pharmacist analyzes the prescription, identifies the Drug Related Problems (DRPs) and resolves the same in consultation with the prescriber and the patient. The goal of pharmacist in pharmaceutical care is to meet the patient's need for appropriate, effective, safe and convenient drug therapy in terms of desired therapeutic outcomes and improved health related quality of life.

Who needs Pharmaceutical Care?

Ideally all patients, who take pharmaceutical products or services, should receive the pharmaceutical care. However due to the time constraints, lack of professional staff, it is difficult to provide pharmaceutical care to all patients. Thus based on the need, patients suffering from chronic diseases such as diabetes, hypertension and asthma, and the patients with poly pharmacy may be prioritized for providing the pharmaceutical care services.

Documentation and monitoring of the care is also an important step in pharmaceutical care process.

DRUG RELATED PROBLEMS (DRPs)

Pharmacotherapy involves both benefits and risks. The risks include the side effects and adverse effects of the drugs while using them to treat diseases. Many researchers observed that, the adverse effects of the drugs may lead to hospitalization, affect the desired therapeutic outcomes, patient's quality of life and increase health care expenditure. The negative impact of the drug therapy may result in morbidity and mortality.

In pharmaceutical care practice, drug related problems are analysed during the treatment and suitable solutions are worked out to minimize or prevent them.

Drug Related Problem (DRP) is defined as "an undesirable event that a patient experience that involves or is suspected to involve drug therapy and that actually or potentially interferes with desired patient outcome".

Drug Therapy Problems in Practice

In 1998, Cipolle had proposed eight categories of Drug Related Problems.

1. Indication without drug
2. Drug without indication
3. Improper drug selection
4. Inappropriate dosage
5. Adverse drug reactions
6. Drug – Drug and Drug – Food interactions
7. Failure to receive drug
8. Non adherence to medication

DESCRIPTION OF DRUG RELATED PROBLEMS

Indication without Drug

When a patient is suffering from an illness and develops a new or worsening of the current situation requires additional drug therapy. For example a patient suffering from Rheumatoid Arthritis using NSAIDs for symptom relief may present symptoms of Gastritis. This situation requires an additional drug such as H_2 blocker Ranitidine or proton pump inhibitor Omeprazole to control the gastritis symptoms. In order to treat a chronic condition such as hypertension, if combination therapy of different mechanisms is required such as use of calcium channel blocker and beta blocker in achieving goal blood pressure. In the management of Tuberculosis along with 4 drug therapy (Isoniazid + Rifampicin + Ethambutol + Pyrazinamide) the patient may be advised to take pyridoxine to prevent peripheral neuropathy caused by Isoniazid.

Drug without Indication

During the course of treatment, prescribers are often enthusiastic to control the signs and symptoms of the disease. In the process of that, patient may be exposed to potent drugs that do not have any medical indication. A drug without suitable indication will pose unnecessary toxicity or side effect to the patient and also forces the patient or payer for additional cost. For example if a patient is diagnosed as asthmatic and advised to take salbutamol inhaler 200 mcg 3 times a day and Budesonide DPI 100 mcg bid. The patient is also prescribed Tab. Pantoprazole 40 mg OD for 15 days. If the patient has not complained any symptoms of gastritis or peptic ulcer disease, use of Pantoprazole can be considered as a drug without suitable indication.

Improper Drug Selection

If a patient is not receiving intended positive outcomes of a prescribed therapy, this may be due to wrong selection of the drug. Unfortunately patients expose to this kind of situation frequently. It is also essential to have a balance between the benefits and side effects of the medicine for desired quality and comfort of the patient's life.

- Any given drug regimen be considered as wrong for a specific patient at a given time if the dosage form is in appropriate (A 55 year old patient with mild angina receiving nitroglycerin patches to be applied on daily basis),
- Contraindications are present (A pregnant woman receiving Isotretinoin 20 mg twice daily for two weeks for acne vulgaris),
- The patient condition is refractory to the drug (a child with otitis media receiving amoxicillin 125 mg thrice daily with a previous history of unsuccessful exposure to the same drug),
- The drug is not indicated for the patient condition or more effective drug therapy is available (For example a patient suffering from chronic asthma is being treated for hypertension with propranolol, the drug for hypertension is being considered as wrong drug because it possess bronchoconstructive property).

INAPPROPRIATE DOSAGE

The best diagnostic techniques, assessment and skills to care for the patients will become nullified if patients are receiving inappropriate doses of potentially effective medications. This may lead to serious and expensive health care problems. Following are the examples of inappropriate dosage.

(a) **Wrong dose:** A two year old child receiving amoxicillin 40 mg orally (40 mg/5 ml) for her first episode of Otitis Media.

(b) **Inappropriate frequency:** A 45 old man with peptic ulcer receiving Omeprazole 20 mg t.i.d.

(c) **Duration inappropriate:** A 15 old boy receiving Amoxicillin 250 mg tid for respiratory tract infection for 3 days.

(d) **Incorrect administration:** The doctor has prescribed Amoxicillin 125 mg/ 5ml tid for respiratory tract infection for 4 year old boy. The medicine bottle comes with a measuring cup. But the mother uses a plastic baby spoon to measure the dose.

Adverse Drug Reactions

The objective of good therapy is to ensure that the patient receives the most effective and safe medication. When it comes to the safety, the most commonly used word is adverse drug reactions. Adverse drug reactions are considered as one of the drug therapy problems that can prevent a patient receiving complete benefit of the therapy. Within the practice of pharmaceutical care, adverse drug reactions are defined as undesirable negative effects caused by the medications that are not predictable based on the dose, plasma concentration and pharmacology of the drug. Following are the common causes for the patients to experience adverse drug reactions.

(a) If the patient receives a drug product which is unsafe.

(b) Patient having a known allergy to the prescribed medicines.

(c) Incorrect administration.

(d) Potential drug interaction leading to an adverse drug reaction.

Example of an Adverse Drug Reaction

A 15 year old patient received Ofloxacin 200 mg b.i.d and paractamol 500 mg t.i.d for fever. After two days of the treatment, the patient experienced bleeding from gums and heamturia. He was immediately taken to the hospital. The doctor has ordered for blood picture. The lab values suggest that the platelet count was 15000. Literature review reveals that multiple doses of Ofloxacin can cause Thrombocytopenic purpura. So this reaction is probably Ofloxacin induced thrombocytopenic purpura.

Drug – Drug and Drug – Food Interactions

Drug – drug and drug – food interactions are considered as one of the important drug therapy related problems. Patient care involves use of multiple medicines to achieve desired therapeutic goals. In the process of that, patient may take two or more medicines at a time. When two or more medicines are taken at a time, patient may experience either a good benefit or no benefit or severe side effects. This situation is resulted due to either pharmacokinetic or pharmacodynamic reason. Pharmacist may identify the potential for drug interactions and frame suitable strategies to minimize them.

For example if a diabetic patient was asked to take ciprofloxacin for cellulites if the patient takes ciprofloxacin as advised by the doctor and also uses antacid which he was taking for his gastritis may lead to potential drug interaction between antacid and ciprofloxacin leading to a therapeutic failure. The mechanism involved in this case is ciprofloxacin requiring acidic environment in the stomach for its absorption. However concomitant use of antacid neutralizes the stomach pH and the absorption of ciprofloxacin will be hampered. To prevent this situation, pharmacist should advise the patient to take antacid after two hours of ciprofloxacin's use.

Failure to Receive Drug

This situation is commonly seen in the hospital set up. Despite the prescriber has ordered the medications for the patient, the duty nurse may fail to administer the drug. This may happen due to heavy work load, altered concentration, change of nurses during the shifts and forgetfulness. In community settings, the patient may not purchase the medicine due to high cost of the therapy or forgetfulness. If patients do not take the intended medicines at the prescribed timings, the patient may not get the desired therapeutic benefits.

Non Adherence to Medication

Compliance represents behaviour of the patient. Any amount of care taken for the diagnosis and giving a prescription will become futile if patient does not take the medicines as per the instructions given in the prescription. Non compliance will lead to therapeutic failure, recurrence of the symptoms or aggravation of the clinical condition and increased cost of the therapy. Cost of the therapy, non availability of the medicine, poly pharmacy, adverse effects and forgetfulness are common causes identified for non compliance. Pharmacist can play a vital role in improving the patient's medication adherence behaviour. Pharmacist can use suitable aids such as drug dosing calendars, use of large, visible print on labels, telephone reminders, and auxiliary directions to explain the appropriate use of the medications to improve the medication adherence behaviour in patients.

SKILLS REQUIRED FOR GOOD PHARMACEUTICAL CARE PRACTICE

In order to provide good pharmaceutical care to the patients, pharmacists are required to possess the following skills.

- Good communication skills.
- Sound knowledge on therapeutics.
- Prescription interpretation skills.
- Maintenance of records.

Good Communication Skills

Patient communication in clinical practice is defined as the dialogue between the pharmacist and the patient for the purpose of obtaining the information needed to assess the patient status and to provide required support and education on drug therapy, diet and life style modification in order to achieve the desired therapeutic outcomes.

In order to have successful patient interaction, pharmacist should possess the qualities like active listening, body language and voice modulation.

Important steps involved in the communication process are,

- Opening the interview
- Setting the stage for good communication
- Obtain complete information
- Control the flow of information
- Closing the interview

After identifying the patient who requires pharmaceutical care, the pharmacist should go through the patient medication record to analyze the potential drug related problems. It is ideal to have the interaction with the patient in a private or semiprivate environment. The interaction should be done in a professional and in a relaxed way. Self introduction with the patient will ease the communication process. It is ideal to use more open ended questions to collect disease related information, medication related information, social life, and attitudes towards the disease management.

Be empathetic towards the patient during the conversation. During the course of discussion it is essential to pay utmost attention to what patient is saying and tailor responses to his or her comments. Provide necessary information regarding medicines, diet and life style modifications to the patient and close the interview with suitable feedback questioning and summing up the information.

Sound Knowledge on Therapeutics

Therapeutics is defined as the application of medication knowledge such as mechanism of action, fate of the drug in the body, dose and dosing schedules, contraindications and drug interactions in the management of diseases. Sound therapeutic knowledge will help the pharmacist to identify potential drug related problems and find suitable strategies to resolve them.

Prescription Interpretation Skills

A prescription is defined as a medication order given by the clinician to treat the patient. In co-morbid conditions, patients may have to take two or more medicines. Before dispensing the medicines, if the prescription is reviewed, pharmacist will be able to identify potential drug related problems and will have the opportunity to discuss the same with the prescriber and the patient to resolve them.

Maintenance of Records

Documentation of the services provided to the patient will act as proof of the Pharmaceutical care practice. With the help of softwares available in the market, pharmacist can develop patient medication records and can use them to update the patient *vs* medication related information as and when required. This ensures the quality of practice and also improves the patient's health.

THE PHARMACEUTICAL CARE PROCESS

A systematic approach to the delivery of pharmaceutical care involves the following steps.

Step **1:** Assess the patient's drug therapy needs and identify actual and potential drug related problems.

Step **2:** Develop a care plan to resolve and prevent the drug related problems.

Step **3:** Implement the care plan.

Step **4:** Evaluate and review the care plan.

A Systematic Approach to the Delivery of Pharmaceutical Care

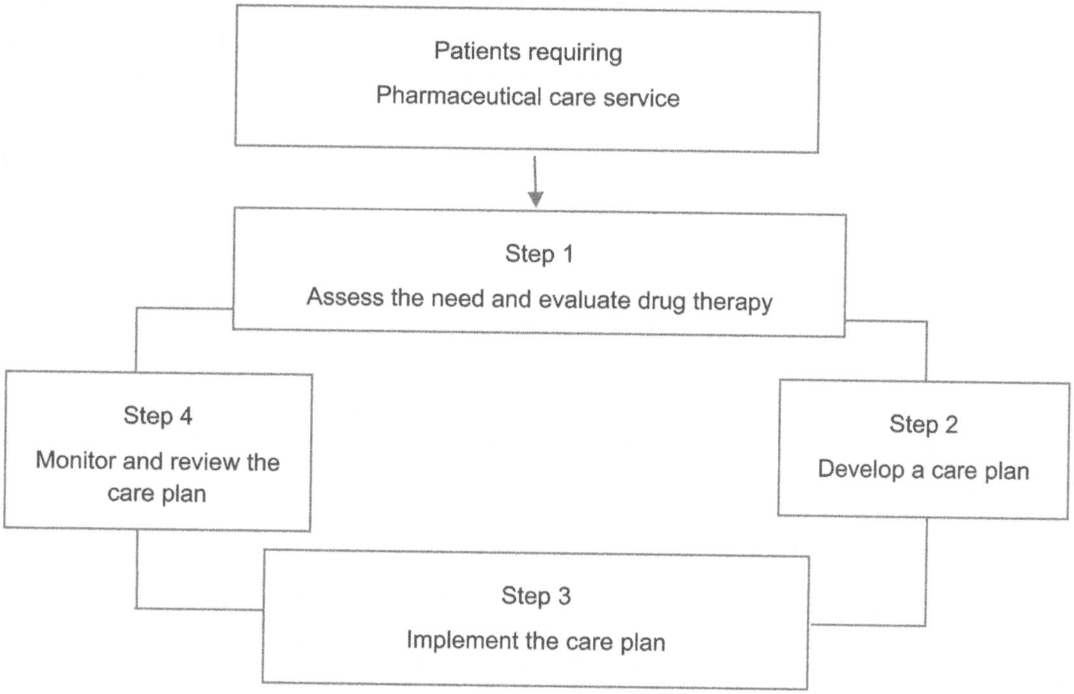

PHARMACEUTICAL CARE STEPS

Step 1: Assess the Patient's Drug Therapy Needs and Identify Actual and Potential Drug Therapy Problems

This is an important step in the pharmaceutical care process. In this step the pharmacist will be able to identify disease related and drug therapy related problems in consultation with the patient and patient's health care provider. In addition, pharmacist may also identify opportunities for health promotion and illness prevention. The pharmacist reviews the patient risk factors like demographic characteristics such as age, gender and weight, relevant medical history and current active medical problem, impairment of organs responsible for drug metabolism and elimination such as liver and kidney, previous history of allergy to any medicines, functional and cognitive factors such as mobility, dexterity and comprehension. This information is generally available in patient medical records or patient case records. Interview with patient or patient's care giver, the pharmacist can collect information on social and environmental factors such as home environment, social drug use and family support, patient's health beliefs including perception of drug therapy and anticipated benefits of the therapy. Pharmacist should assess the response to current drug therapy, manifestation of allergies if any, complexity of the regimen and use of devices such as inhalers, rota halers and insulin pens etc.

Step 2: Develop a Care Plan

Care plan is an agreement between the pharmacist and the patient regarding the medication use management. During the care plan, the pharmacist in consultation with patient understands the drug therapy needs, identifies potential and actual drug related problems, develops strategies to resolve them and establish patient specific goals in achieving the desired therapeutic outcomes. For example, if a patient has developed an unpleasant effect after the use of certain medicine, the care plan includes listing the patient problem(s), the drug involved in causing the problem and assessing the association between the drug and the patient's problem.

Step 3: Implement the Care Plan

After deciding the care plan, the pharmacist will make suitable and acceptable interventions in consultation with both prescriber and the patient. The pharmacist will document all the interventions made regarding the therapy in patient's case notes for prescriber perusal and acceptance.

Step 4: Monitor and Review the Care Plan

This is a follow up stage in the care plan. Follow up consists of scheduled interaction with the patient by the pharmacist to assess the outcomes of the proposed interventions such as the recommended care plan has produced the desired outcomes or not or resulted any other new problems.

Pharmaceutical Care Services

As per the definition by Strand *et al.*, pharmaceutical care services includes all the services such as drug dispensing, drug information, patient counseling, drug therapy monitoring and health screening services. All the activities can be done in a spacious community pharmacy manned by a trained practicing community pharmacist.

BARRIERS TO IMPLEMENT PHARMACEUTICAL CARE

The pharmaceutical care service is an outcome oriented and provider specific practice in the interest of patient care. However due to various reasons, the community pharmacists may not show interest to provide pharmaceutical care services. These reasons are considered as barriers. The barriers may be pharmacist based or pharmacy specific. The pharmacist based barriers are lack of time, increased work load, lack of knowledge and training to provide the service, lack of assertiveness, poor communication skills, non legalization of the services and lack of remuneration and an assumption that the patient care is the doctor's responsibility.

Pharmacy based barriers are inadequate space and facilities, inadequate aids for providing pharmaceutical care to the patients.

CONCLUSION

Pharmaceutical care is a patient oriented approach in identifying, resolving and preventing drug therapy problems. The entire process includes assessing patients' drug therapy needs, developing a care plan, implementing the same and reviewing the care plan to assess the achievement of pharmaceutical care objectives and if necessary review and revise the care plan. In order to provide efficient pharmaceutical care, the provider should have sound therapeutics knowledge, effective communication skills, prescription interpretation skills and effective documentation.

KEY POINTS

- Pharmaceutical care is responsible provision of drug therapy in order to achieve the desired therapeutic goals and improve patients' quality of life.
- Good communication skills, sound knowledge in therapeutics, prescription interpretation skills are the essential qualities for a pharmacist to provide effective pharmaceutical care.
- A systematic approach to provide pharmaceutical care is to assess the patient's drug therapy requirements, analyze drug related problems, and resolve them in consultation with the prescriber and the patient.
- Lack of knowledge, training and non legalization of the services, inadequate facilities are the identified barriers for providing pharmaceutical care.

SUGGESTED READINGS

1. Hepler CD and Strand L.M (1990). Opportunities and responsibilities in Pharmaceutical Care. *Am J Hosp Pharm* **47:** 533-545.
2. Robert J Cipolle, Linda M Strand and Peter C Morley. Pharmaceutical Care Practice. McGraw Hill Publication.
3. Seedhouse D (1995). Reforming Health care: The Philosophy and practice of International health reform, Chichester, Wiley, England.

CASE STUDY

Mrs. JS a 55 years old lady diagnosed as type 2 Diabetes Mellitus and was put on Glibenclamide 5 mg. Her relevant medical history includes hypertension for the past one year and was on Atenolol 50 mg CD, Osteoarthritis and Angina. Her current drug therapy includes

Naproxen 500 mg BID

Glyceryl Trinitrate 2.5 mg BID oral

Haloperidol 0.25 mg OD at bed time

Let us try to identify the drug related problems in the above prescription order and indicate whether they are actual or potential problems.

In order to assess the drug related problems, patient should be enquired about her past disease related and medication related history.

Upon enquiry, the patient told that she is having osteoarthritis for last 5 years and she used to take regularly OTC NSAID from the local chemist and as she developed gastritis and heart burning, she visited her General Practitioner, who prescribed Omeprazole 20 mg OD and Naproxen 500 mg BID. After a weeklong treatment, she has become normal and she continues to take Naproxen for her osteoarthritis. Few months later, she had developed severe chest pain. On consultation, her GP informed that she has developed angina and put her on Glyceryl trinitrate 2.5 mg BID oral and Haloperidol 0.25 mg at bed time. After few months, in her routine examination, her blood pressure was found to be 145/95 mmHg. After a week, the doctor repeated the B.P examination and found her B.P as 150/100 mmHg and she was prescribed with Atenolol 50 mg OD.

Step 1: Drug therapy problems identified in this case

Inappropriate drug: For long term therapy of osteoarthritis, Naproxen is not an appropriate drug. If Naproxen is to be continued, cytoprotection is required in elderly patients. Paracetamol and life style modifications may be appropriate in Mrs. JS.

Requiring medication: As Mrs. JS developed angina, she may have chances to suffer from ischemic problems. Low dose aspirin may be highly beneficial in this patient. But the patient is not receiving the Aspirin.

Drug without valid indication: Review the need for Haloperidol. No specific indication is observed in this patient for Haloperidol. Chances of Haloperidol induced side effects are high in the elderly patients.

Step 2: Develop a care plan to resolve and prevent drug therapy problems

After identifying the drug therapy problems, a discussion with the patient and the doctor may be initiated and a care plan may be developed to resolve or prevent the identified drug therapy problems. Not all patients reach to this situation. Patients who are with multiple diseases and multiple drugs may be the right candidates for providing pharmaceutical care. In order to analyze and provide the care services, it is essential that, pharmacists should have the necessary resources such as text books (Text book of Pharmacotherapeutics, Text book of Clinical Pharmacy), compendia (Drug information hand book, Pharmacist hand book) and data bases such as Micromedex.

Step 3: Evaluate and review the care plan

Actual outcomes are evaluated in relation to the therapeutic objectives to determine whether drug therapy problems have been resolved. If expected outcomes are not achieved, it is essential to review the care plan and if necessary modify the care plan to achieve the best possible therapeutic out comes. In case, if old problems have been resolved and new problems have come up then plan should be reworked to resolve the new problems.

Step 4: Learning Activity

Identify 3 patients with different diseases in your own practice and follow the above steps using the documentation form provided along with this chapter. Analyze your strengths and weaknesses and improvise upon your weaknesses in consultation with a clinical pharmacist and your preceptor.

Step 5: Description of actual therapeutic outcomes

Status	Definition
Resolved	Goals achieved, therapy completed
Stable	Goals achieved, continue same therapy
Improved	Progress being made and continue the same therapy
Partial Improvement	Progress being made, minor adjustments are required
Unimproved	No progress but continue with the same therapy
Worsened	Decline in health, adjust the therapy
Failure	Goals not achieved, probably need new therapy
Expired	Patient died while receiving the therapy

Appendix

Primary Care Medication Review Form

Patient Details:

Patient ID:

Name: Age:

Gender: Male/Female

Height: Weight: BMI:

Smoker: Non-Smoker: Ex-smoker:

Blood Pressure: Blood sugar: FBS/RBS

Address:

Tel: Mobile:

General Practitioner's Name:

Address:

Tel: Mobile:

Medical History

Date	Signs and symptoms	Diagnosis

Current Drug Therapy

Drug name inclusive of OTC medications	Date started	Date stopped	Drug related problem if any	Action taken or initiated

While Reviewing the Medications Ask Yourself,

- Is the therapy appropriate?
- Are the doses prescribed appropriate?
- Are there any potential untreated conditions?
- Is there any more cost effective alternative?
- Are there any potential drug-drug interactions?

Pharmaceutical Care Plan

Date	Desired outcome	Proposed action	GP response	Patient outcome

CHAPTER 3

PRESCRIPTIONS

LEARNING OBJECTIVES

- Define prescription
- Know various parts of prescription
- Understand drug related problems in prescriptions
- Know about dispensing labels and filling procedure

Prescription filling is one of the responsibilities of the pharmacists. Thus it is essential for the pharmacists to know about various parts of a prescription, health care professionals those are eligible to write the prescriptions, and the procedure to label and fill the prescriptions. The concept of 'prescription' goes dates back to the beginning of the history. Earliest prescriptions were found in 2700 B.C by Sumerians who lived between Tigris and Euphratus rivers. Early prescriptions were given for herb based medicines requiring mixing, steeping or grinding. Modern prescription medicines are formulated using plant or chemical ingredients. So long as there are medications, a writing system will exist to give directions for preparation and usage.

Modern prescriptions are actually "extemporaneous prescriptions". In Latin (*ex tempore*) "Extemporaneous" means the prescription is written on the spot for a specific patient with a specific ailment. This is distinguished from a non-extemporaneous prescription which is a generic recipe for a general ailment. Modern prescriptions are evolved with the separating role of the pharmacists from that of the physicians. Today the term "extemporaneous prescriptions" is reserved for "compound prescriptions" which requires the pharmacist to mix or "compound" the medication in the pharmacy for the specific needs of the patient. Present days, due to the availability of the readymade dosage forms by pharmaceutical companies, pharmacists' compounding activity has become obsolete. In modern days, prescription refers to a list of medicines to be dispensed to the patient.

DEFINITION

In majority of the countries, both medicine and pharmacy professions are regulated by the government and professional bodies. A prescription is a communication mechanism to patient is also regulated and considered as a legal document. A prescription is a written or computerized order from a prescriber directing the pharmacy to compound and or dispense the medicines for patient's use. Regulations of a respective country may define what a prescription should constitute, the contents and the format (including the size of the paper) and how prescriptions should be handled and stored by the pharmacists. Some countries allow the faxed or phone prescriptions containing the same information.

In some countries the preprinted prescription contains two signature lines: one line indicates "dispense as written" printed underneath; the other line suggests "substitution permitted". Some have a preprinted box "dispense as written" for the prescriber to check off (but this is easily checked off by anyone with access to the prescription). In few countries, the protocol for the prescriber is to handwrite one of the following phrases: "dispense as written", "DAW", "brand necessary", "do not substitute", "no substitution", "medically necessary", "do not interchange". In some countries different codes may be used. For pediatric prescriptions, it is essential to write the age and weight of the child. Prescriptions often have a "label" box. When written, the pharmacist is instructed to label the medications. When not written, the patient only receives instructions for taking the medications and no information about the prescription itself.

PARTS OF PRESCRIPTION

Currently two types of prescriptions are given to the patients. One is the conventional hand written prescription and the other one is the computer generated prescription, which are commonly given in corporate hospitals.

Often patients bring variety of prescriptions to the community pharmacies such as medication name written overleaf of the bus tickets, small piece of paper, or on currency notes. These are not considered as prescriptions. A valid prescription should possess the following parts.

1. Superscription
2. Inscription
3. Subscription
4. Signa

1. **Superscription:** The superscription "Rx" means "take" in effect, "I want this patient to have the following medications." This symbol had originated in medieval manuscripts as an abbreviation of the Latin verb *recipe*, the imperative form of *recipere*, "to take" or "take thus". Literally, the Latin word *recipe* means simply "Take" and medieval prescriptions invariably began with the command to "take" certain materials and compound them in specified ways. Today, when a medical practitioner writes a prescription beginning with "Rx", he or she is completing the command. Folk theories about the origin of the symbol ℞ note its similarity to the Eye of Horus, or to the ancient symbol for Zeus or Jupiter, (♃), gods whose protection may have been sought in medical contexts.
2. **Inscription:** The inscription is heart of the prescription. Inscription lists the names and quantities of the medications to be used. Whenever there is doubt

regarding the name of the medication or the dose mentioned, or duration of the treatment, the pharmacist should consult the doctor for clarification and corrections. This act not only ensures a good rapport with the doctor but also minimizes the dispensing errors.

3. **Subscription:** The subscription follows the inscription and is that part of the prescription that gives directions to the pharmacist.
4. **Signa:** The signa, should not to be confused with the prescriber's signature. This is the part of the prescription that gives the directions to the patient. This portion is preceded by the abbreviation **"Sig"** which is **Prescriber Signature Block.** Finally, the prescriber signature block, located at the bottom of the form, **must** contain a legible signature of the prescriber with date, as well as the prescriber's full name, designation, address including the registration number and contact phone number.

Prescription Number 0012	OP No: 0200908125			
Mrs. Geetha Gowda 45 yr # 692, MIG KHB Colony, Kalpavriksha Nagar, Mysore -7				
Medications	**AM**	**Noon**	**Evening**	**PM**
R_x				
1. Tab. Amodep AT (30)	**1**	**0**	**0**	**0**
2. Tab. Diapride Forte (30)	**1**	**0**	**0**	**0**
3. Cap. Becosules (30)	**0**	**1**	**0**	**0**
4. Tab. Eliwel 12.5 mg (30)	**0**	**0**	**0**	**1**
Dispense as prescribed, **Single filling only**	**Dr. K. Karthik Reddy M.D** **General Physician** **Regd. No. KMC 1290** **Date:**			

Fig. 3.1 Model Prescription

Who are Eligible to Write Prescriptions?

Legally qualified and registered medical practitioners (MBBS, MD, MS) are only eligible to give prescriptions to their patients for managing the illnesses. In some countries, certified nurse may also issue prescription with prior permission or the verbal instructions from the clinician. In some countries, licensed certified physician assistants, optometrists and clinical pharmacists are also eligible to write the prescriptions. However, medical students are not eligible to give the prescriptions.

PRESCRIPTION HANDLING

Before dispensing the medications, it is essential to ensure that the prescription received is bonafide one from an authorized prescriber and the person brought the prescription is a bonafide patient. Prescriptions brought in a piece of paper or on empty spaces of cigarette boxes, or an empty medication strip, should not be dispensed. Once filled the prescription should not be refilled unless instructed by the prescriber.

Pharmacist should study the prescription carefully and make sure that the drug prescribed is reasonable, that its amount or dosage is realistic in consideration with the patient's age, and that the quantity of the medication is practical. For example, a prescription given for 20 Alprazolam tablets, warrants further inquiry. In the process of verification, if a discrepancy, an ambiguity, or an incompatibility is observed in the given prescription, it is appropriate to consult the prescriber. At the same time, patient should not be allowed to suspect that anything is amiss. Pharmacist should never fill a prescription that is not understood or that he or she feels is incorrect. Prescribers will appreciate if pharmacist consults them politely for clarifying the doubts regarding the prescription given by them.

If a prescription is found correct in all respects, an undivided attention is required to fill the prescription. Most mistakes are made when the pharmacists are interrupted while doing so or are trying to accomplish more than one task at a time. During the process of filling a prescription, the label on the carton box or the container should be verified at least three times. Initially, the label should be read when the medication box is taken from the shelf. Then it should be read again when the strips are removed from the container. And finally, label on the container should be read before it is returned to the shelf. By following these three verification steps for each prescription filling, possibility of making a prescription error is minimized. While dispensing, pharmacist should never substitute the prescribed medicines without the permission of the doctor.

PRESCRIPTION LABELING

Prescription labeling is an important task in filling the prescriptions. Prescription labeling helps the patient to take the medications in right quantity, at right time for the advised length of period. Improper labeling misguides the patient. The label should possess information about the name of the patient, age, gender, name, dose of the medication, and its usage instructions to the patient, details of the prescriber with the phone number and dispenser details etc. Directions to the patient regarding the medication use should be given in layman language. Other information that may be attached on the prescription container is "Shake Well before Use" or "For External Use Only".

<table>
<tr><td colspan="2">Mrs. Geetha Gowda 45 yr
692, MIG, KHB Colony, Kalpavriksha Nagar, Mysore -7</td></tr>
<tr><td colspan="2">Tab. Amodep AT 30 Tabs
(Atenolol 50 mg + Amlodipine 5 mg)
Take one tablet after the breakfast. Take the tablet at same time every day for best result.</td></tr>
<tr><td>Prescribed by
Dr.Karthik Reddy

Date:</td><td>Dispensed by
T.Venu
Dispensing Pharmacist
Sai Nihar medicals</td></tr>
</table>

Fig. 3.2 Dispensing Label

After dispensing the medications, the pharmacist should fix a seal "DISPENSED" on the prescription to prevent the misuse of the prescription for refilling unless otherwise indicated by the prescriber as number of refills permitted such as ONE or TWO. It is also important to convey the message to patients to destroy the unused medicines for safety reasons.

Filing of Prescriptions

In some countries pharmacists are expected to file the dispensed prescriptions for various reasons. As a legal document, the regulations mandate the pharmacist to archive the original paper prescription in the pharmacy. Often the patients cannot take the original prescription with them. Some jurisdictions may entitle patients to a copy. The retention period varies but can be as long as ten years. In case the pharmacy is sold out or closed permanently for any reasons, the pharmacist is expected to return the prescriptions to the patients or to nearby pharmacy.

CONVENTIONS TO AVOID CONFUSIONS IN INTERPRETING THE PRESCRIPTIONS

To avoid the ambiguity and misinterpretation of the prescriptions, prescribers have developed many conventions for prescription-writing. These include:

1. **Careful use of decimal points to avoid ambiguity**
    - Avoiding unnecessary decimal points: A prescription will be written as 5 mL instead of 5.0 mL to avoid possible misinterpretation of 5.0 as 50.
    - Always using zero prefix decimals: E.g., 0.5 instead of .5 to avoid misinterpretation of .5 as 5.
    - Avoiding trailing zeros on decimals: E.g., 0.5 instead of .50 to avoid misinterpretation of .50 as 50.
2. "mL" is used instead of "cc" or "cm^3" even though they are technically equivalent to avoid misinterpretation of 'c' as '0' or the common medical abbreviation for "with"

(the Latin "*cum*"), which is written as a 'c' with a bar above the letter. Further, cc could be misinterpreted as "c.c.", which is an uncommonly used abbreviation for "take with meals" (the Latin "*cum cibo*").

3. Directions written out in full in English.
4. Quantities given directly or implied by the frequency and duration of the directions.
5. Where the directions are "as needed", the quantity should always be specified.
6. Where possible, usage directions should specify the time at which the medicine should be taken such as 7 am, 3 pm, 11 pm rather than simply writing the frequency (three times a day) and especially with relationship to meals for orally consumed medication.
7. Using pen with permanent ink while writing the prescription.
8. Avoiding unspecified ***prn*** or "as needed" instructions–instead, specific limits and indicators are provided e.g., "every 3 hours prn pain".
9. For refills, the minimum duration between repeats and number of repeats should be specified.
10. Providing the indication for all prescriptions even when obvious to the prescriber, so that the pharmacist may identify possible errors.
11. Avoiding units such as "teaspoons" or "tablespoons".
12. Writing out numbers as words and numerals ("dispense #30 (thirty)")
13. The use of apothecary/avoirdupois units and symbols of measure -- pints (**O**), ounces (℥), drams (ʒ), scruples (℈), grains (**gr**), and minims (♏) -- is discouraged to avoid the confusion. For example, the abbreviation for a grain ("gr") can be confused with the gram, abbreviated g, and the symbol for minims (♏), which looks almost identical to an 'm', can be confused with micrograms or metres. Also, the symbols for ounce (℥) and dram (ʒ) can easily be confused with the numeral '3', and the symbol for pint (O) can be easily read as a '0'. Metric equivalents should always be used to avoid the errors.
14. The use of the degree symbol (°), which is commonly used as an abbreviation for hours (e.g., "q 2-4°" for every 2-4 hours), should not be used, since it can be confused with a '0'. Further, the use of the degree symbol for primary, secondary, and tertiary (1°, 2°, and 3°) is discouraged, since the former could be confused with quantities (i.e., 10, 20 and 30, respectively).

PRESCRIPTION ABBREVIATIONS

Following abbreviations are commonly used in the prescriptions. It is important for the pharmacists to know these abbreviations.

Abbreviation	Latin	Meaning
aa	ana	of each
ad	ad	up to
a.c.	ante cibum	before meals
a.d.	auris dextra	right ear
ad lib	ad libitum	use as much as one desires; freely
admov.	admove	apply
agit	agita	stir/shake
alt. h.	alternis horis	every other hour
a.m.m.	ad manu medicae	at doctors hand
a.m.	ante meridiem	morning, before noon
amp		ampule
aq	aqua	water
a.u.	auris utraque	both ears
b.d./b.i.d.	bis in die	twice daily
bol.	bolus	as a large single dose (usually intravenously)
B.S.A		body surface areas
cf		with food
D.A.W.		dispense as written (i.e., no generic substitution)
d.t.d.	dentur tales doses	give of such doses
h.s.	hora somni	at bedtime
mane	mane	in the morning
od	oculus dexter	right eye
p.c.	post cibum	after meals
p.m.	post meridiem	evening or afternoon
p.o.	per os	by mouth or orally
p.r.	per rectum	by rectum
PRN,	pro re nata	as needed
stat	statim	immediately
wf		with food (with meals)
f.i.d	Ter in die	Three times a day
g.i.d	Quarter in die	Four times a day

KEY POINTS

- Prescription is a written medication order given to a patient with a purpose to treat the patient.
- Legally qualified and registered medical practitioners are only eligible to write prescriptions.
- A valid prescription should possess superscription, subscription, inscription and Signa.

- While the dispensing the prescription, the pharmacist should check the correctness of the prescription and fill the prescribed medications appropriately.
- For any clarification regarding the dispensing instructions, the pharmacist should never hesitate to consult the prescriber.

SUGGESTED READINGS

1. A Text Book on Prescription writing and pharmacy. By Bernard Fantus. Chicago Medical Book Company, USA.
2. Ansel H (2010). *Pharmaceutical Calculations*. 13th edition, Philadelphia. Lippincott, Williams, and Wilkins.
3. Skills and Procedures for Medical Assistants. Thomson Delmar, Cengage Learning publishers, 2004, USA.

CHAPTER 4

PATIENT COUNSELING

LEARNING OBJECTIVES

- Know the definition of patient counseling
- Identify the patients who require counseling
- Understand the outcomes of patient counseling
- Know various counseling stages
- Appreciate the counseling barriers and find strategies to overcome them

INTRODUCTION

Health care includes medical care, pharmaceutical care, and nursing care. In medical care, clinicians diagnose the disease, analyzing the signs and symptoms, lab results and radiological results prescribe the medications to treat the disease. Patients take medicines regularly if they are informed about how important their medicines in bringing down the signs and symptoms. Due to heavy patient load, often prescribers find difficulty in providing medication related information to the patients.

Due to lack of medication usage information, patients may tend to forget taking the medication or misuse the medications. Pharmacists by virtue of their Pharmacotherapeutics knowledge are in the right position to give suitable advice to the patients regarding safe use of medications. World Health Organization (WHO) and International Pharmaceutical Federation (FIP) identified patient counseling as one of the important professional responsibilities of the pharmacists.

Definition

Patient counseling is defined as "providing information to the patient or patient's care giver regarding the disease, medication, diet and life style modifications in layman language to achieve the desirable therapeutic outcomes". The information may be given verbally and complimented with written information leaflets.

Outcomes of Effective Patient Counseling

- Patient will understand the importance of the prescribed medication in management of the disease.
- Improved medication adherence.
- Achieving the desired therapeutic goals.
- Reduced incidence of adverse effects and unnecessary health care costs.
- Improved quality of life.
- Improved professional rapport between the patient and pharmacist leading to an improved patient patronage to the pharmacy.

Effective patient counseling is not simply providing the information. The timing and organization of information are very important to improve the patient's understanding and motivation to follow the instructions given during the counseling session.

Often in community pharmacies, pharmacists are busy in filling the prescriptions and patients are in hurry to receive the medication. Every patient receiving medication should know about how to use them. But in busy practice it may not be feasible. Following guidelines may be used to identify the patients, who need counseling.

Patients Requiring Counseling

- Patients, or their care givers confused about the use of medicines
- Patients with impaired sight or hearing
- Illiterate patients
- Patients whose profile shows a change in medications or dosing
- New patients or those receiving a medication for the first time
- Parents receiving medication on behalf of the children
- Patients receiving medication in mechanized devices such as inhalers, rotahalers and medications with special storage requirements, complicated directions and with significant side effects

Patients who should be Counseled at Regular Intervals

Following patients generally require counseling at regular intervals

- Asthmatic patients
- Diabetic patients
- Patients taking 4 or more medications
- Patients using devices containing medication
- Epileptic patients
- Patients with skin complaints
- Patients misusing drugs
- Patients who are terminally ill

Art and Science of Counseling

The counseling act is considered as an opportunity for information exchange between the pharmacist and the patient. Pharmacist is an expert on drug therapy, but patients are experts on their daily routines. Patients' understanding about the illness and the treatments, problems in taking the prescribed medicines are the important concerns during the counseling. Each of these points needs to be assessed for an effective counseling. For an effective patient counseling, the pharmacists should update their medication knowledge and should possess required communication skills.

United States Pharmacopoeia (USP) and other health care institutions worked on science and technology of patient counseling. USP has listed about 174 counseling items that can be used during the counseling process but finalized about 30 counseling items that can be used based on the practicality. Following patient counseling items may be useful during the counseling process. The list may help the pharmacists to use various counseling items in different situations. The Pharmacist is expected to review the case record and analyze the drug therapy before the counseling session.

Counseling Item Check List

As per United States Pharmacopeia there are more than 90 counseling items which may used to educate the patients. However in Indian set up following counseling items may be sufficient for counseling purpose.

1. ***Introduce yourself:*** It is important for the patients to know that they are speaking with the pharmacist. They may be reluctant to ask questions or express concerns with a salesman. So Pharmacists should greet the patient, and state their name: "Hello, I'm Prasad, your pharmacist. May I help you". This creates a good beginning for successful professional relationship.
2. ***Identify to whom you are speaking:*** If you are talking to the patient directly you may give the desired information to the patient directly, but if you are speaking to the patient's representative you must be careful in providing the information as they have to pass the information to the patient. In third party communication written information is ideal. Pharmacists may call patients if they believe that the information needs to be communicated directly to them.
3. ***Ask if the patient has time to know about their medicine:*** Patients visiting community pharmacies are often will be busy in taking their medications and going home. If patients do not have time to listen, the information provided will be ineffective. In such situation, an information leaflet may serve the purpose or if the patient is interested, patient may be asked to come at a mutually convenient time.
4. ***Explain the purpose/importance of the counseling session:*** Before beginning the counseling session, the pharmacist should tell them that they may know about disease, medicines, diet and lifestyle modifications. Ensure them that during the counseling session they can also clarify their doubts.
5. ***Ask the patient what did the physician told about the disease and the medicines prescribed:*** Ask the patient what did his/her doctor told about the disease and

medicines. This will help the pharmacist to assess the patient's knowledge and tailor the information as per the patient requirement.

6. ***Prior to providing information, ask the patient if he/she has any concerns:*** Often, patients will not vocalize concerns about the drug(s) they are about to take or the condition the doctor is treating unless they are asked. It is important to address these concerns for a fair discussion.

7. ***Listen carefully and respond with appropriate empathy:*** Listening to the patient is very important for an effective counseling session. Careful listening gives an opportunity for the pharmacist to understand the patient's awareness about disease and medicines. Showing empathy to patients will improve the patient's confidence on pharmacist and this will help in improving the patient's attention towards the counseling.

8. ***Tell the patient about the name, indication, and route of administration of the medicine:*** This step often takes place after filling the prescription and dispensing of medications to patients. Telling patients about the name of the medicine helps them to identify it. This is especially important in case of an emergency (e.g., a child ingesting it or in overdose). Stating the indication reinforces the diagnosis and creates confidence in the appropriateness of the therapy. Explaining about the route of administration prevents the patients to wrongly administer the medication. E.g.: Chewing or taking the pessary through oral route. It should not be assumed that printing this information on the label will solve the problem. Many patients who cannot read may not know about the route of administration and those who read also often ignore the information on the label.

9. ***Inform the patient about the dosage regimen:*** Patients should be informed about their dosage regimen in order reinforce what the doctor has instructed. Dosage regimen also should be informed when the patient is taking the medicine for the first time. For example an instruction "Take one tablet after meals" may prompt some patients to take their medications more than the intended times per day. The diabetic patients may take meals more frequently in small quantity. If the information is correctly given, patient will stick to the instructions.

10. ***Ask the patient if he/she has any problem in taking the medication as prescribed:*** This is an important question that is seldom asked by any healthcare provider. Often cost of the therapy, non availability of the medication, regimen complexity, and adherence are the common patient related problems. Research studies have corroborated that the complexity of the dosage regimen can greatly affect the patient's compliance. Once-a-day dosing generally achieves rates of compliance greater than 80%, while four-times-a-day dosing reduces compliance to below 40%. Selecting an economical brand, working with the physician to change the medication to a less complicated dosing schedule will resolve.

11. ***Incorporate the medication regimen in to the patient's daily routine:*** To improve the medication adherence, patients should be advised to incorporate the medication into their daily routine. As they plan the day, if medications are also incorporated in their

daily routine planner, chances of missing the doses will be very less. Keeping alarm in their mobile or maintaining a pill box will help the patient to improve the adherence.

12. ***Tell the patient how long it will take for the drug to show an effect:*** Patients should be clearly informed about the duration the medication takes to show the therapeutic effect. If patients are not well informed about this, the patient may stop taking the medicine or double the dose.

13. ***Tell the patient how long he/she might be taking the medication:*** Patients need to have a reasonable expectation of how long they will need to take the medication. This helps them get into a "mind set" of compliance. It also helps to eliminate unrealistic expectations. Moreover, it gives patients a chance to express concerns about the length of treatment.

14. ***Tell the patient when he/she is due for a refill (and the number of refills needed):*** Patients need to plan in order to be compliant, and this information assists them in doing so. The information may be given in the form of a verbal contract. The pharmacist should say, "Mrs. Rekha, the doctor has given you a 30-day supply. Therefore, may I see you on June 30th for next refill?" By doing this, the pharmacist helps the patient to know when to come back for the next refill.

15. ***Emphasize the benefits of the medication:*** Pharmacists should make every effort to support the chosen therapy and tell patients about the benefits of the treatment before they discuss potential side effects. This not only helps to put side effects in perspective, but it also promotes patient confidence in the therapy. Lack of confidence in the chosen therapy will result in a higher incidence of noncompliance.

16. ***Discuss major side effects of the drug:*** It is very important to discuss about the major side effects with the patients. While discussing about this information, pharmacist should be very specific with information regarding side effects. Pharmacist should emphasize on what side effects may be experienced? When they will subside? If the side effects are non tolerable what to do? etc., should be discussed with the patients. It is possible that some patients do not want to know about any side effects, and some may want to know all possible side effects. Pharmacists should develop a flexible approach to the dissemination of information. Leaflets are an excellent way to provide patients with additional information.

17. ***Point out that additional, rare side effects are listed in the information sheet:*** An information sheet summarizing the facts about the medication should be given to the patient at the end of the counseling session. Emphasize the rarity of some of the side effects listed, and encourage the patient to call if he/she has any concerns about these.

18. ***Use written information suitably to support the counseling process:*** For literate patients, written information has been shown to reinforce verbal instructions given by the pharmacist. The patient can also go through the leaflet in leisure to recall the pharmacist's instructions. In addition, it can be used to promote more effective counseling. Written information may be given to patients to look over while their prescriptions are being dispensed. This can prepare patients to ask better questions and help the pharmacist to talk less.

19. ***Discuss precautions (e.g., activities to avoid) and beneficial activities (e.g., exercise, decreased salt intake, diet, self-monitoring):*** It should not be assumed that the physician has discussed these things with the patient. Ask patients what they have been told, and discuss if necessary.

20. ***Discuss drug-drug, drug-food, and drug-disease interactions:*** Patients generally are not aware that other medications, foods, or diseases may interfere with the drug(s) they are taking or affect the condition for which they are being treated. For example, a patient with high blood pressure should be told to ask the pharmacist before taking any medicines for coughs or colds. The patient should also be told why these precautions are necessary.

21. ***Discuss storage recommendations, ancillary instructions (e.g., shake well, refrigerate):*** Many patients still store their medications in medicine cabinets in the bathroom or kitchen-probably the worst places in the house to keep medicines because of humidity and heat. Give general storage recommendations for all medicines, and specific storage recommendations (e.g., refrigeration) and ancillary instructions to the patient.

22. ***Explain to the patient in precise terms what to do if he/she misses a dose:*** Actual times of day and specific examples should be used to make this clear. The patient should then be asked, for example, "What will you do if it is 5:00 p.m in the evening and you realize you have missed your noon dose?" if the patient says yes to this question, inform him/her not to repeat the same. If the patient realizes that he/she has missed the dose at the time nearing to the next dose, he or she may be encouraged to skip the old dose and take the next dose but the same should not be repeated.

23. ***Check for further understanding by asking the patient to repeat back additional key information:*** To fully assess whether the patient understands the dosage regimen, you could say, "Mrs. Lakshmi, sometimes information can be a little confusing. Just to be sure I was clear, could you tell me how you are going to take your medication?" The same may be done with side effects, storage conditions, etc. To better control the time this takes, more specific questioning might be useful: "Mrs. Lakshmi, what time will you take your first dose?" Correct answers should be praised and incorrect information should be corrected. Praising has been shown to reinforce compliance.

24. ***Check for any additional concerns or questions:*** The counseling session may have raised additional questions or concerns. The pharmacist should ask if this is so and listen respectfully and carefully to what the patient has to say.

25. ***Advise patients to always check their medicine before they leave the pharmacy:*** This helps to familiarize patients with their medicine and makes them a partner in ensuring an error has not been made. The pharmacist should say, "Please always check your medicine before you leave the pharmacy. If you have any questions or problems about the way it looks, please notify me. I don't intend to make any mistakes, but it's good to be cautious. You are the final check. By doing this you are emphasizing that this is a partnership in which the patient also has responsibilities.

26. ***Use appropriate language throughout the counseling session:*** On occasion, pharmacists use language that is unnecessarily confusing (e.g., hypertension rather

than high blood pressure; GI instead of gastrointestinal or stomach). Many patients will not say they are confused because they do not want to appear stupid. If you detect any confusion, it may be helpful to ask, "Have I said something that has confused or concerned you?" Language that is simple and understandable promotes compliance.

27. ***Maintain control of the counseling session:*** A great deal of information needs to be covered in order to counsel the patient effectively. Concerns take time to address. Therefore, keep superfluous conversation to a minimum. "Small talk" is helpful to start the counseling session, but it needs to be brief and simply serve to break the ice.

28. ***Organize the information in an appropriate manner:*** Generally speaking, the most important information should be provided at the beginning of the counseling session and repeated at the end. In addition, support of the drug should precede side effects. This checklist has been formulated to reflect the recommended organization of the counseling session.

Follow up to Determine how the Patient is Doing

Follow-up care is a good way to:

1. Differentiate your services
2. Let patients know you are concerned about them
3. Increase your refill prescription business

Very few healthcare providers offer follow-up care. Yet abundant evidence indicates that patients tend not to get their refills on time and some never return at all. Advise patients that not refilling chronic medications on time places them at risk for further problems, and offer reminders about refills. Follow-up care should be done voluntarily and should be as flexible as possible.

Keep in mind that some patients may not want it. Patients should be enrolled in a follow-up care program and given options as to how they receive it. For example, some may prefer a telephone call, while others may prefer a postcard, a letter, or a fax. The more flexible you can be in providing this service, the more likely it will work.

Written Patient Information Leaflets

When patients are busy and to complement the verbal information provided during the counseling, information leaflets play vital role. Patient may use information leaflets to update the information and can read at their convenience.

Counseling Area

The patient should be counseled in a semi-private, or private, area away from other people and other distractions, depending on the medication(s). The patient should perceive the counseling area as confidential, secure and conducive for discussion. This helps to ensure both parties focus on the discussion, and minimizes interruptions and distractions. This also provides an opportunity for patients to ask questions they may be hesitant to ask in public.

Communications Skills required for Effective Counseling

Patient counseling is an art as well as science. Knowledge regarding medicines and diseases and skills to communicate effectively make the pharmacist as a good counselor. Counseling skills can be improved over a period of time by practice. The counseling process uses verbal and non-verbal communication skills.

Verbal Communication

Skills include language and paralinguistic features such as tone, volume, pitch, and rate of speech. Para linguistics, or the way we say words, accounts for 40% of how a message is received so the way in which we speak has an impact on patient's understanding.

Language: While speaking with patients, use simple language and avoid using unnecessary and difficult medical words. If possible, communicate the information in patient's own language.

Tone: Tone of our voice is very important during the course of counseling. Changes in the level and range of pitch convey information about the feelings and attitudes of the person speaking. During the counseling' the tone of the voice should be caring and reassuring.

Volume: Many people speak with wide variations in volume, depending on the situation, and where and to whom they are speaking. Ideally counseling should be conducted in a quiet, private setting where it is unnecessary to raise one's voice. Although it may be necessary to speak more loudly to patients with a hearing problem, most deaf patients gain more benefit if the speaker moves closer, and directs their voice towards the patient's ear.

Speed: Clarity of our communication depends on our rate of speech. Patients may be reluctant to interact with a pharmacist who speaks quickly because they may feel the pharmacist is too busy. This may happen if the pharmacist is nervous or is uncertain about the information being given. In contrast, the person who speaks too slowly may lose the interest of the listener. For good verbal communication, the pharmacist should present clear, relevant messages in a logical sequence, and at a speed which gives the patient time to think about what is being said. This will help the patient to understand and remember the concepts more easily.

Non-verbal Communication

Includes body language such as the movement and position of the head, limbs, and body, and other aspects such as whether the pharmacist is dressed in a professional manner. During any interaction approximately 50% of the way a message is received comes from body language. Aspects of nonverbal communication skills include proximity, touch, eye contact, facial expressions, and head movements, gestures with hands and body postures.

Proximity: This refers to the distance that people maintain between themselves during the counseling process. This space has been classified into four zones; intimate (45 cm or less) personal (45 cm - 1.2 m), social (1.2 m - 3.6 m) and public (more than 3.6 m). Generally counselors or health care professionals use intimate or personal proximities.

Eye contact: The amount that people look at one another during conversation varies depending on whether they are speaking or listening. Listeners look at the speaker more often and for longer periods of time. For cultural reasons or personal reasons such as timidity, sadness or depression some people may avoid looking into the counselor's eyes.

Facial expression: These can be used during counseling to demonstrate empathy towards the patient. Head movements such as nodding, hand gestures, and body postures also can be used to advantage.

INCENTIVES FOR COUNSELING

Every professional expects some incentive for the services provided to their clients. Pharmacists also expect a legible incentive for the services provided to their patients. Since patient counseling is not legalized in India, following may be the incentives pharmacists may anticipate for providing the counseling.

- Professional satisfaction
- Increased customer patronage to the pharmacy leading to an increased sale.

Barriers for Patient Counseling

Following are the barriers identified for not happening of the patient counseling in India. The barriers are classified in to the following groups.

- Patient based barriers
- System based barriers
- Provider based barriers

Patient based barrier: Counseling happens only when patients show interest in receiving the information. If they are in hurry to reach home it is very difficult to talk to them. Gender difference, language difference, and literacy are the identified patient based barriers.

System based barriers: Lack of reimbursement due to non-legalization of patient counseling, lack of adequate space and trained staff and the busy hours are considered as system-based barriers.

Provider based barriers: Provider is the Pharmacist. In India, majority community pharmacies run by pharmacists having Diploma in Pharmacy qualification. Their knowledge and their commitment towards counseling are inadequate. Lack of interest, lack of time, lack of knowledge, lack of confidence, lack of training are identified as pharmacist based barriers.

Strategies to Overcome the Counseling Barriers

To overcome the patient based barriers, following strategies can be implemented.

- Using multimedia materials
- Pictograms
- Oral or written information
- Compliance aids

- Follow up schedules
- Audiovisual tapes
- Tailoring prescription instructions

Legalization of the patient counseling, introduction of counseling fee and continuous professional development programs are the important strategies to improve the counseling activity in pharmacies.

KEY POINTS

- Patient counseling is considered as an important professional responsibility of the pharmacists.
- Effective counseling improves medication adherence behavior in patients and results in positive health outcomes and improved health related quality of life.
- Based on the situation and the patient's condition, appropriate counseling items may be employed from the counseling items inventory.
- Suitable verbal and non verbal communication skills are important to make the counseling more effective.
- Legalization of patient counseling, implementation of professional fee, continuous professional development programs for patients, use of pictograms, information leaflets will help in overcoming the counseling barriers.

SUGGESTED READINGS

1. Bruce Berger. Communication Skills for Pharmacists: Building Relationships, Improving Patient Care.
2. Harvey M. Rappaport *et al.,* (1994). The Guidebook for Patient Counseling. Lancaster, Pennsylvania: Technomic Publishing Company.
3. Melanie J. Rantucci. Pharmacists Talking with Patients: A Guide to Patient Counseling. Wolter Wilkinsson Publication.
4. Tindall, William N, Robert S. Beardsley, and Carole L. Kimberlin (2003). Communication Skills in Pharmacy Practice (fourth edition). Baltimore, Maryland and Philadelphia, Pennsylvania : Lippincott William & Wilkins 2003.

USEFUL WEBSITES

1. https://www.ihs.gov/healthcommunications/documents/toolkit/Tool9.pdf
2. www.ashp.org/s_ashp/docs/files/BP07/Org_Gdl_PtEduc.pdf
3. www.cuhk.edu.hk/med/ans/Good%20Communication.pdf
4. www.snpha.org/Files/Forms/316/**Patient**%20**Counseling**%20Module.pd

CASE STUDIES FOR COUNSELING

CASE STUDY I

Mr. JR is a 45 year old, moderately built bank officer who recently consulted his physician for his nose bleed and early morning dizziness, and increased frequency of micturition. His doctor advised for Fasting Blood Sugar (FBS), and Post Prandial Blood Sugar, Blood Urea Nitrogen and serum creatinine. His blood pressure was recorded as 152/92 mm Hg. His FBS found be 165 mg/dl (90-110 mg/dl) and PPBS found to be 225 mg/dl and BUN is 40 mgldl and Serum Creatinine is 1.4 mg/dl.

Mr. JR was given the following drugs.

Rx

Tab. Enalapril maleate 5 mg oneOD

Tab Glimepiride 1mg one BD Tab Metformin 500 mg one BD

What counseling points should be given to Mr. JR?

Discussion

From the case records, we can find that Mr. JR's problems are Hypertension and Diabetes Mellitus. He was put on antihyperensve medication, and oral hypoglycemic agents. Whether the patient can spare some time for counseling should be asked and with patient's consent, the counseling session can be started.

First by using open ended questions, his hobbies, past medication details, awareness about his disease, drugs and diet and life style changes should be assessed. Based on his understanding counseling information to be given can be planned. Later, information on his medication such as name of the drug, dose, duration of the therapy, possible side effects and storage should be given.

For patients with hypertension and diabetes mellitus, diet and life style modification are important. In life style modifications, information on foot care, nail care and aerobic exercises should be told to him. Cessation of alcohol and cigarette smoking are important.

Information about hypoglycemic shock, such as signs and symptoms, suitable solutions such carrying raw sugar, or sugar candy should be told to him. At the end of the session his understanding should be assessed with feed back questioning. His final doubts may be allayed and he should be advised when to return back to the pharmacy for refilling of his prescription.

Medication usage Information

Enalapril Maleate: This medication lowers and brings increased blood pressure to normal. The recommended dose of Enalapril is 5 mg. It should be used once in a day at your own fixed time like may be after the lunch. Sometimes this drug may cause dry cough or change in the taste. Inform to your doctor or pharmacist about it for necessary remedy

Glimepiride: This drug is given to reduce your elevated blood sugar level and brings it to normal. Take this drug twice daily, before morning and evening meal.

Metformin: This drug is given to control your elevated blood sugar levels. Take this drug twice daily after morning and evening meals.

When you are on blood sugar reducing drugs, some times suddenly the blood sugar level may fall down below the normal. This is called as hypoglycemia. The symptoms of this condition are, sweating, increased heart rate, and confusion. When you experience such effects, eat a small sugar candy, or a spoonful of sugar. If medications are not taken correctly as prescribed, blood sugar level may not be brought down to the control levels and may lead to damage of heart, kidney, eyes, blood vessels, nerves and feet.

Diet: A normal Indian diet with little modifications may be a suitable diet. In the diet consider eating more vegetables containing fiber and green leafy vegetables. Eat less of nuts, cereals, pulses, fruits and meat products. Avoid eating sweets, honey, jams and jellies.

Exercise: With the help of the doctor, a suitable exercise plan can be made. The most ideal one is a brisk walk for about 3 km in 30 minutes.

Foot care: Diabetic patients should check their feet regularly and keep them clean. Suitable diabetic footwear should be used to prevent foot ulcers.

CASE STUDY 2

Mr. C 1 aged 35, presented the prescription to the community pharmacy which was given at the time of discharge from the local hospital. Mr. CN's asthma was first detected when he was in high school and during a football match. After the initial treatment Mr. CN was free of symptoms. Recently the disease has become worse and required hospital admission. Present prescription contains the following medication.

Rx

Salbutamol MDI 200 g four times a day

Beclomethasone MDI 200 g Four times a day

Prednisolone tablets 10 mg every morning

Ranitidine tablets 150 mg twice daily.

Give the stepwise counseling to Mr. CN on his medication.

Mr. CN case is an acute exacerbation of asthma. Many asthma patients become exacerbated due to the poor medication adherence, knowledge about the disease, triggering factors, symptomatology and management techniques.

Before providing the necessary counseling points, it is essential to assess the knowledge, awareness and practice of the patient with respect to the disease and medication. Based on the knowledge and awareness, patient should be educated about the inflammation process of the asthma, time taken to relieve the inflammation, risk factors, medications prescribed to relieve the congestion and how long they should take medication.

Medication Usage Information

Salbutamol 200 mcg MDI: This medication is given to open up the air passages of lungs. The recommended dose is 200 mcg. In order to get 200 mcg, the patient is required to take two puffs with one minute gap.

Beclamethasone 200 mcg MDI: This medication is corticosteroids used to prevent the symptoms of asthma. When used regularly every day, this medication decreases the number and severity of the attacks. This medication work by preventing certain cells in the lungs and breathing passages from releasing substances that causes the symptoms. This inhaler gives 200 mcg per puff. So inhalation of one puff gives required dose.

When the patients are on inhalers, they should be educated about the inhaler usage technique.

The recommended technique for the proper use of the MDI

- Remove cap
- Shake the container
- Breath out gently not fully
- Hold inhaler up right and place lips around the mouth piece or 2 finger width from mouth.
- Start to inhale slowly immediately before actuation
- Actuate inhaler while continuing to inhale
- Inhale completely and hold breath for 10 seconds
- Wait one minute
- Repeat the treatment if more than one inhalation prescribed

For inhaled steroids, rinse mouth with water or mouth wash and expel Contents.

Prednisolone: This medication is used to suppress the allergic and inflammatory process in bronchial asthma. This medication may be taken after the breakfast to prevent gastric irritation.

Ranitidine: This medication is given to reduce the gastric irritation caused by Prednisolone. This medication is required to be taken morning and evening before meals.

Providing a patient information leaflet about asthma can strengthen the information provided by the counselor.

CHAPTER 5

PATIENT INFORMATION LEAFLETS-READABILITY AND DESIGN

LEARNING OBJECTIVES

- Understand the importance of readability criteria in developing information leaflets
- Know about various readability formulas
- Appreciate the lay out and design characteristics of an Information leaflet
- Appreciate the counseling barriers and find strategies to overcome them

INTRODUCTION

Communication skills play very important role during the patient counseling. Patient counseling is a two way communication process to address the disease, medication, diet and lifestyle modification related issues. The counselor may empathetically identify and understand the information gaps with the patients and accordingly provide the required information. Many patients will be visiting the pharmacies and will be busy in collecting the medicines and leaving the pharmacy. In such situations, information leaflets serve as useful tools to know the disease or medication related information. Many patients can read these information leaflets at their convenience and understand the medication usage related information. Sometimes patients may use these information leaflets to update their knowledge. Many published research articles have corroborated the usefulness of patient information leaflets during the counseling process as an aid to compliment the verbal instructions.

Pharmaceutical producers often supply information regarding their products as package inserts. However these package inserts are hardly found useful to the patient due to strong medical jargons used in preparing the text and are more focused for the use by health care professionals. In such situation, information leaflets prepared in layman language will help the patients to know about their disease and medication. The prime objective of providing information leaflets to the patients is to assist the patients in filling the knowledge gaps and help them to update their understanding about the disease and medication related information at their convenience.

Educational background of the patients generally ranges from illiterate to university education. In English speaking country like United States of America, researchers have reported that, most of the Americans of 14 years age or older cannot read better than seventh grade student. Eighth to Ninth grade level is frequently reported as standard reading level for the overall American population. In India with 50% of literacy rate, average Indian adult population can comprehend the written English of below 5th grade only. When written communications are aimed at such patients, lot of care is required in framing the sentences. The comprehensibility of such leaflets can be assessed by the readability assessment formulas.

A readability formula is a simple method to predict the reading grade level required to comprehend the written materials. Readability formulas are predictive instruments and provide an index of probable reading difficulty. In assessing the readability, actual participation of the reader is not required. The formulas measure the structural difficulties of written materials such as vocabulary and sentence structure but fail to evaluate other factors related to readability such as conceptual difficulty, organization of the material, content or reader characteristics like interest in the subject, motivation, life experiences or patient knowledge about the subject. As on date, more than 40 different formulas have been published to evaluate the readability. Most of the readability formulas are derived statistically and consider only language variables such as word complexity and sentence length. Apart from the readability, layout and design characteristics of the leaflet are also equally important to increase the appeal of the leaflet. An attractive designed document generates interest in the reader. Kitching and Baker Able's guidelines are the best example guidelines in designing the information leaflets.

In the present chapter some important readability formulas, readability calculation methods, and layout and design guidelines are presented for the benefit of the readers and researchers interested in developing the information leaflets.

READABILITY TESTS AND THEIR APPLICATION

Comprehension is influenced by the difficulty of reading materials. During the past 3 decades, many systematic procedures have been developed to add objectivity to the evaluation of reading materials. There are two methods to evaluate the readability. One is based on the length of words and sentences and the other one is based on the predictability of words in the reading passage. The first method is exemplified by a number of reading formulas. The second uses a simple procedure of deletion from standard word lists. Neither method is considered ideal, but however have enough of relationships with readability to justify their evaluative use.

READABILITY FORMULAS

Various readability formulas have been published in the last three decades. However the most important and useful formulas are **SMOG Formula, Fog formula by Gunning, Fry Readability graph, Spache Grade – Level Score, Flesch Reading Ease formula,** and **Flesch Kincaid Grade level formula.**

1. **SMOG Formula:** The SMOG formula, published in 1969 by McLaughlin determines the reading grade level necessary to fully comprehend written material. This formula is based on average word length and has a standard error of prediction of 1.5 grades and takes less than 15 minutes to calculate the reading difficulty. It is simple and fast to use without losing accuracy. The SMOG formula is based on 100% comprehension, whereas the other formulas are based on 50% to 75% comprehension. Thus it is a more conservative predictor of readability since it gives scores two grades higher than score predicted by other formulas.

   General Guidelines for using the SMOG formula:

   (a) A Sentence is defined as a string of words, punctuated with a period, an exclamation point, or a question mark.

   (b) Proper nouns, with three or more syllables should be counted

   (c) Abbreviations should be read as unabbreviated.

   (d) Verbs ending in 'ed' or 'es' that add a third syllable to the word should not be included

   (e) Hyphenated words are considered as one word.

   (f) Numbers spelled out or written as numbers should be pronounced to determine if they have three or more syllables

   Procedure to calculate readability score of written text containing 30 or more sentences

   - Count 10 consecutive sentences near the beginning, 10 in the middle and 10 near the end of the text to be evaluated.
   - From these 30 randomly selected sentences, count every word with three or more syllables.
   - Calculate the square root of the number of words with three or more syllables. This is done by finding the nearest perfect square and taking its square root.
   - Add a constant of three to calculated square root

   Procedure for a text of less than 30 sentences

   Count all the words containing 3 or more syllables

   - Count the number of sentences
   - Find the average number of words with three or more syllables per sentence as below

$$\text{Average} = \frac{\text{Total number of words with 3 or more syllabus}}{\text{Total number of sentences}}$$

- Multiply this average by the number of sentences short of 30
- Add this value to the total number of words with three or more syllables
- Calculate the square root and add the constant of three

The given table illustrates an example of SMOG Formula

Example:

Number of words with 3 or more syllables	– 47
Nearest perfect square root	– 49
Square root	– 07
Add constant	– 03
SMOG Reading grade level	7 + 3 = 10

The SMOG reading grade level 10 suggests that, the reader must reach tenth standard to understand the written material

2. **FOG Formula by Gunning:** The FOG formula is one of the easiest methods for calculating grade level readability, because it is based on a short sample of 100 words and does not require counting all syllables or applying many rules.

   Method of Analysis

   1. Count 100 words in succession (W). If the piece is long, take several samples of 100 words each from throughout the selection and average the results.
   2. Count the number of complete sentences. If the word mark falls in the middle of a sentence, include this sentence in the count. This count becomes 'S' in the formula below.
   3. Divide the words (100) by the number of sentences (S)
   4. Count the number of words having three or more syllables (A), but do not count
      (a) verbs ending in 'ed' or 'es' that make the word have third syllable,
      (b) capitalized words, or
      (c) combination of simple words, such as butterfly.
   5. Apply the formula to calculate the grade level

$$\mathbf{GL = (W/S + A) \times 0.4}$$

Where GL is the grade level, W is the number of words (usually 100), S is the number of sentences, and A is the number of words having 3 or more syllables.

Advantages: It is useful for checking the readability of informal materials, such as study guides, work sheets and tests between the levels of grade 4 and college.

3. **Fry Readability Graph:** The Fry readability graph may be useful for a quick estimation of the grade level readability of materials from grade 1 to college. This method uses a few simple rules applied to the Readability graph (figure 1) to determine the overall readability of a wide range of materials.

   Method of Analysis

   1. Select 100 word samples from the beginning, middle, and end of a book or pamphlet. Do not count proper nouns as part of the 100-word count.
   2. Count the number of sentences in each sample of 100 words, estimating to the nearest tenth of a sentence for partial sentences
   3. Average the sentence counts of the three samples
   4. Count the number of syllables in each sample
   5. Average the syllable counts of the three samples
   6. Plot the sentence count and word count on the graph to determine the grade level

   Advantages: It overlaps with applications of the Flesch and Fog formulas, but the reader may find it especially useful for books, long pamphlets or brochures.

4. **Spache-Grade Level Score:** The Spache method is designed to determine the grade level of materials written for grades 1 to 3 and may be useful, in designing or evaluating materials for children. It requires the use of a list of common words in the form of Dale's list of 769 familiar words. The methodology for readability determination is very similar to the Flesch method.

   Method of Analysis

   1. For short selections, test the entire selection. For longer selections, test at least three randomly selected samples of 100 words each.
   2. Determine the average sentence length (a) by counting the number of words in the sample and dividing by the number of sentences. Count as a sentence each independent unit of thought that is grammatically independent, i.e., if in end in punctuated by a period, question mark, exclamation point, semi colon or colon. If the 100 word mark in the sample falls often the midpoint of a sentence, count this sentence as part of the sample
   3. Count the number of words not on the Dale list (b) with the following exceptions
      (a) Count a word only once, even if it appears several times
      (b) Do not count first names
      (c) Do not count as different words plural forms made by changing endings
      (d) Do not count adjective and adverb forms as different words.

4. Apply the formula

$$GL = 0.141\ a + 0.086\ b + 0.839$$

where GL is the grade level, 'a' is the average sentence length, and 'b' is the number of words not listed on the Dale list of 769 familiar words.

Advantages: This formula is useful for assessing the readability of children books like comics, and storybooks.

5. ***Flesch Reading Ease Formula:*** The Flesch method develops data to predict reading difficulty without the need for validation by sample of readers. The grade levels and degrees of reading difficulty is determined by the formula have been validated repeatedly over 30 years of use. The analysis is based on the average sentence length (in words) of selected samples and the average word length measured by syllables per 100 words of the sample. These two variables are combined to yield a Flesch Reading Ease Score (FRE).

Method of Analysis

1. For short pieces, test the entire selection. For longer pieces, test at least three randomly selected samples of 100 words each. Do not use introductory paragraphs as part of the sample. Start each sample at the beginning of a paragraph.
2. Determine the average sentence length by counting the number of words in the sample and dividing by the number of sentences. Count as a sentence each independent unit of thought that is grammatically independent. i.e., if end is punctuated by a period, question mark, exclamation point semi colon or colon. In dialogue, count speech tags (E.g., "he said") as part of the quoted sentence
3. Determine the word length (WL) by counting all the syllables in the sample as if reading the words aloud. Divide the syllables by the number of words in the sample and multiply by 100.
4. These indices are then applied to the formula to compute the reading ease.

$$RE = 206.835 - 1.015\ SL - 0.846\ WL$$

where RE is the reading ease scores, SL is the average sentence length in words, and WL is the average word length measured as syllables per 100 words.

Interpretation of Flesch Reading Ease Score

Reading Ease	**Description of style**
90 –100	Very easy
80 –90	Easy
70 –80	Fairly easy
60 –70	Standard
50 –60	Fairly difficult
30 –50	Difficult
0-30	Very difficult

Advantages: This method is useful for determining the readability level between grade 5 and college graduate.

5. **Flesch-Kincaid Grade Level:** Flesch Kincaid grade level score rates texts of US schools. For example, a score of 8.0 means, that an eighth grader can understand the document. For most standard documents, a score of approximately 6.0 to 8.0 is aimed.

   The formula for the Flesch-Kincaid Grade level score is (0.39 * ASL) + (11.8 * ASW) – 15.59.

   where,

   ASL = Average sentence length (the number of words divided by the number of sentences)

   ASW = Average number of syllables per word (the number of syllable, divided by the number of words)

   Both Flesch Reading Ease Score formula and Flesch Kincaid grade level formulas are available in Microsoft word. In order to assess the readability scores of a document, the simple procedure is, type the document in word. Click on tools, and then move the cursor on to the spelling and grammar and click. Later go to option and click on show readability statistics, press OK. Then press Ignore all to see the readability statistics.

Patient information leaflet – Lay out and Design Guidelines

Appropriate Layout and Design of a leaflet improves the patient's acceptance. Many guidelines were published to show model information leaflets. In 1990, Kitching recommended the following guidelines for content and layout to prepare a patient information leaflet with good acceptance by reader.

1. Line in a PIL should be 50-89 mm long
2. There should be a 2.5mm separation between two lines
3. Unjustified lines are easier to read
4. Serif type of letter face is easy to read
5. Letter type should be of at least 12 points
6. Indenting the first line of a paragraph increases reading speed
7. Titles all in capitals are harder to read than lower cases
8. Italics impair comprehension
9. Points should be positive rather than negative
10. Headings should stand out in a different type or extra space
11. Arabic numerals (1,2) are easier than roman (I, II etc)
12. Numbers are easier as numerals – '9' is easier than 'nine'
13. Highlighting by colour or boxing is not helpful
14. Pictures are helpful for complex maneuvers (E.g., Inserting suppositories or eye drops) but others may distract.

Basara and Juergens scored leaflets for print size, graphics, colour printing, amount of white space and paper quality. Baker Able also developed useful guidelines for the layout and design of leaflet similar to Kitching, Baker Able also stressed on length of line (50-80mm) separation between lines, (>2.8mm) unjustification of lines, Serif type face, type size (>12 point) indenting of first line, lower case titles, words in italics, (0-3 words) positive advice, standard headings, numbers in Arabic, boxed tent (0-1 Box). Apart from these specifications, Baker Able added three more important criteria in the design of leaflet. They are, number of colours used, (4 Colours) amount of white space (% of page area, Eg. Cm2, >40%) and paper quality (>90 gsm)˙ Baker Able Leaflet Design (BALD) criteria is used commonly to assess the layout and design of various patient package inserts (PPI).

CONCLUSIONS

Average Indians' English comprehension capability may be less than 5th grade level. Most of the pharmaceutical companies supply package inserts for Registered Medical Practitioners use or laboratory use. Many pharmaceutical formulations like, topical preparations, suppositions, aerosol preparations in mechanical devices, and medications in novel drug delivery systems require suitable instructions to the patient for proper usage of medication. Thus, time has come for the manufacturers to prepare and supply patient information leaflets to the patients in simple English and the local language. While preparing the information leaflets, it is very important to consider the readability and design of the leaflet. The readability formulas and layout and design guidelines discussed in this chapter are more accepted by international pharmaceutical manufacturers, pharmacy associations, and pharmacists.

KEY POINTS

- Patient Information Leaflets (PIL) compliments the counseling process and helps the patients to understand and update the medication related information at their convenience.
- Majority Indians comprehend the written material of less than 5th grade. Thus it is very essential to prepare information leaflets with easy comprehension.
- Although more than readability formulas are available, Flesch Readability ease Score is a standard formula even adopted by Microsoft Word.
- Baker Able Leaflet Design criteria is commonly used to calculate the layout and design score.

SUGGESTED READINGS

1. Eaton ML and Holloway RL (1980). Patient comprehension of drug information. *Am J Hosp Pharm.* **37:** 240-3.
2. Fry E (1968). A readability formula that saves times. **11:** 512-6, 575-8.
3. G.H Mc Laughlin (1969). SMOG rating, A new readability formula. *J Reading* **12:** 639-646.
4. G.R Karle (1974-75). Assessing readability. *Reading research Quarterly* **10:** 62-102.
5. Gunning R (1952). The technique of clear writing. New York: McGraw Hill Co. 29-39.
6. John S Dowder (1996). Consumer information affects us all. Australian Prescriber **19(2):** 30-31.
7. Kitching J B (1990). Patient information leaflets – the state of art. *J R Soc Med.* **83:** 298-300.
8. Lisa Ruby Basara and John P Juergens (1994). Patient Package inserts readability and design. *American Pharmacy.* **NS34:** 48-53.
9. Louise Mallet and William J Spruill (1988). Readability evaluation of nine patient drug education sources. *American Pharmacy* **28:** 33-36.
10. Spadaro DC, Robinson LA and Smith LT (1980). Assessing the readability of patient information materials. *Am J Hosp Pharm.* **37:** 215-21.
11. Stuart J Baker (1997), who can read consumer product information. *Aust J Hosp Pharm.* **27:** 126-131.

FRY GRAPH FOR ESTIMATING READABILITY LEVELS

The sample point shown in the graph indicates the readability of thep content is seventh grade. The average number of syllables is 141 and average length of sentence is 6.3.

Average number of syllables for 100 words

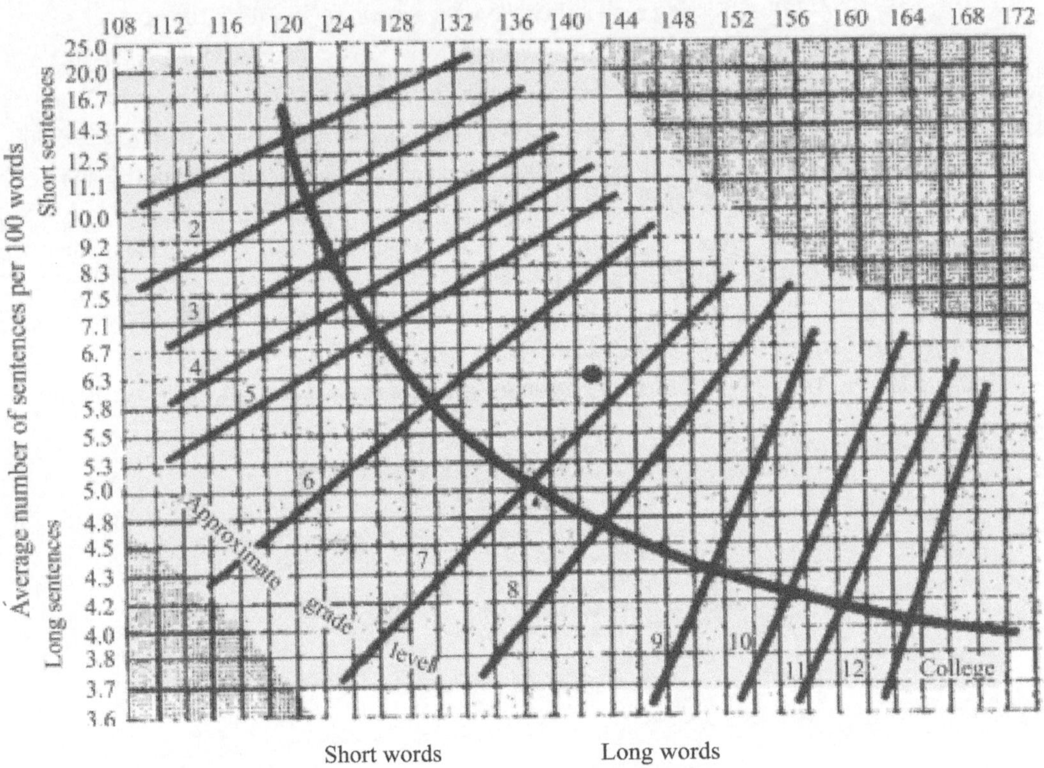

Fig. 5.1

CHAPTER **6**

HEALTH SCREENING SERVICES

LEARNING OBJECTIVES

- Appreciate the importance of health screening services in patient care.
- Know the technique of checking blood pressure.
- Record capillary blood glucose using glucometer.
- Assess the lung function using peak flow meter.

Health screening services are the patient care services that are provided by the pharmacists in community pharmacies. Health screening services play an important role in early detection of the diseases, and thereby early treatment and prevention of the complications of the disease. Community pharmacists can also involve in monitoring and managing the chronic disorders like hypertension, diabetes mellitus, hyperlipdemia, asthma. Monitoring refers to observation and in some cases intervention of the disease condition after the diagnosis and treatment, which helps to assess and improve the outcome.

The role of community pharmacists in offering the screening services is not to overtake the role of the physician but to provide the patients an opportunity to check the improvement in their health as a part of the disease management. Number of studies published in Australia and in other countries has assessed the usefulness of health screening services in community pharmacies. A study conducted by Snella *et al.* assessed the role of pharmacists in screening elderly and patients with risk for diabetes, hypertension, and dyslipidaemia (blood pressure, blood glucose and lipids) in pharmacies and in non-health care settings. Nearly 900 patients with risk factors were screened and detected new cases of diabetics (3%), hypertension (3%) and dyslipidemia (10%) and upon referral to the GPs, they confirmed the diagnosis and initiated the treatment.

Trained community pharmacists can implement and provide the health screening services at the community pharmacy. The Pharmaceutical Society of Australia (PSA) *Professional Practice Standards* described the standards for provision of health screening and monitoring the patients. Adherence to these standards will ensure that pharmacists who are implementing screening programs deliver a professional, reproducible, and high quality services. These standards include six main criteria as follows:

- Proper use and maintenance of the equipment

- Receiving adequate training and improving the competence of personnel involved in the screening process.
- Documented procedures for recording the results
- Safety issues regarding body fluids handling
- Explanation of results
- Monitoring of screening outcomes and referral processes.

Health screening services may be offered to individuals who are at high risk for a specific disease. The procedures for the following health screening services are explained in detail.

- Measuring blood pressure for hypertension
- Checking blood glucose levels for diabetes mellitus
- Calculation of body mass index (BMI)
- Peak expiratory flow rate (PEFR) by peak flow meter for asthma

MEASUREMENT OF BLOOD PRESSURE

A person is considered as hypertensive when on two or more consecutive measurements if diastolic blood pressure is more than 90 mmHg and the systolic blood pressure is more than 140 mmHg. Poor control of blood pressure may cause target organ damage like cardiac, cerebro vascular, renal, and ocular and may become a cause for death.

Table 6.1 Classification of Blood Pressure for Adults Aged ≥ 18 Years: 7th Report of Joint National Committee (JNC 7)

JNC 7 Blood Pressure Category	SBP (mmHg)	and/or	DBP (mmHg)
Normal	< 120	and	< 80
Prehypertension	120-139	or	80-89
Hypertension:			
Stage 1	140-159	or	90-99
Stage 2	≥ 160	or	≥ 100

Pharmacists as a part of health care system, taking initiatives to measure the blood pressure of the people with risk will have the following advantages.

- New hypertensive patients can be detected.
- Can help patients to monitor their blood pressure and observe the usefulness of medications.
- Motivate the patients to improve medication adherence behavior.
- Can prevent hypertensive consequences.
- Can minimize the work load of general practitioner.

Generally an individual who is above 18 years of age can have his or her blood pressure measured. Only qualified and well trained persons are advised to measure the blood pressure.

Blood pressure is measured to detect or to diagnose hypertension. The instrument used to record blood pressure is Sphygmomanometer.

Following techniques are practiced for accurate measurement of blood pressure using sphygmomanometer:

- Patients should be seated quietly for at least 5 minutes in a chair (rather than on the exam table) with their backs supported and their arms bared and supported at their heart level.
- Patients should be refrained from smoking or ingesting caffeine during the 30 minutes preceding the measurement.
- Correct measurement of blood pressure requires the use of a cuff that is appropriate to the size of the upper right arm.
- The bell of the stethoscope should be lightly placed over the brachial artery pulse, proximal and medial to the cubital fossa, and below the bottom edge of the cuff (i.e., about 2 cm above the cubital fossa).
- The cuff should be inflated to 30 mmHg above palpated systolic blood pressure (SBP) and deflated at a rate of 2 to 3 mmHg/second. Both SBP and diastolic blood pressure (DBP) should be recorded. The first appearance of sound (phase 1) is used to define SBP. The disappearance of sound (phase 5) is used to define DBP in adults.
- Two or more readings separated by 2 minutes should be averaged. If the first two readings differ by more than 5 mmHg, additional readings should be obtained and averaged.
- Elevated blood pressure must be confirmed on repeated visits before characterizing an individual as having hypertension.
- The blood pressure measured should be provided in verbal and written form and advice to consult a physician if there is high blood pressure.

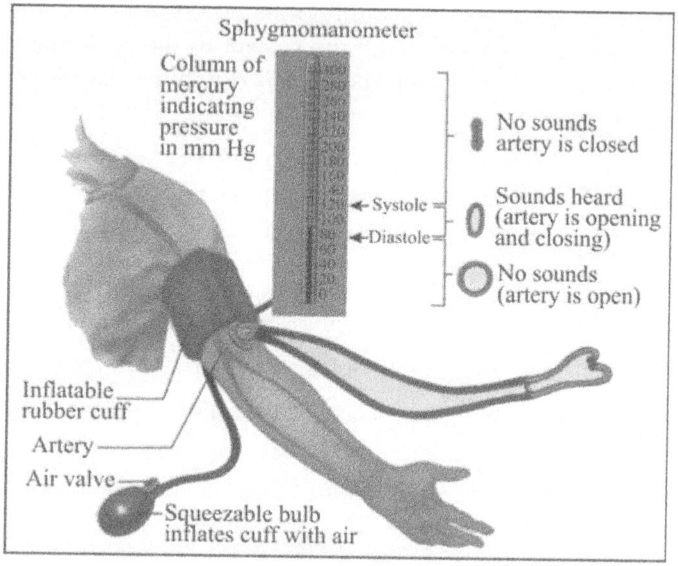

Fig. 6.1 Procedure for Measuring Blood Pressure

Patient Referral form to Refer the Patients to GP/ Consultant for Further Management

Patients recorded to have elevated blood pressure on two consecutive occasions, should be referred to a GP or to a consultant. Format for the referral is given below.

Patient Referral Form
To, Date: Dr. ....
Patient's Name: Age: Gender: Symptoms B.P (using Sphygmomanometer):
Referred By: Name of the Pharmacist: Pharmacy Name Seal & Signature

MEASUREMENT OF CAPILLARY BLOOD GLUCOSE

Blood glucose measurement within a pharmacy can provide valuable information in identifying the individuals with abnormal blood glucose levels. It helps the individual with diabetes and unable to perform his/her own blood glucose monitoring. Blood glucose measurements in community pharmacies should not be used to initiate or alter the treatment. Pharmacist may send a written report through the patient to the physician for further follow up only. In consultation with the prescriber, the pharmacist can counsel the patient regarding the management of the disease.

Measurement of Capillary Blood Glucose (CBG) has become simple with the recently introduced Glucometers. The Glucometer manufacturers made them very simple and user friendly and even patients can measure their CBG without any difficulty.

Who should have blood glucose measured?

Individuals who could benefit from the screening of blood glucose include

- Patients who are expressing anxiety about the development of diabetes mellitus
- Patients' hyperglycemia was controlled by either diet alone or by oral hypoglycemic drugs.
- Individuals who are diabetic and require regular blood glucose monitoring for evaluating the drug therapy.

- Individuals showing symptoms of diabetes such as poly urea, poly phasia, tiredness and weight loss etc.

Blood glucose screening should not be performed by pharmacists on

- Persons under 18 years of age unless requested by doctor.
- Persons with visible evidence of infection on fingers and nails.
- Immunocompromised individuals including persons who are on immunosuppressant drugs.

How to measure blood glucose levels?

To measure blood glucose, a device called Glucometer is required. Various models of glucometers are available in the market produced by different manufacturers. Glucometers function on calorimetric principle. For measuring the blood glucose levels, a glucometer's strip is used. This Glucometer strip possess a hallow place or an identified place, where a blood drop should be placed.

The blood reacts with the reagent present in the identified space and color change is detected by the Glucometers. Before measuring, the Glucometer should be placed in quite and comfortable place. Insert the strip in to the device. This will turn on the machine. Compare the strip code with the code number shown on the screen. If both are different, set the code in the machine using the button.

Sterilize the finger with cotton swab containing an antiseptic agent. Prick the finger with the safe disposable lancet and place the drop of blood on the strip at the loading place. The machine gives the result within 5 to 30 seconds.

Blood Glucose Measurements and Recommendations

Category	Result mg/dl	Recommendation/interpretation
Non diabetic fasting	< 80	Diabetes is unlikely
Non diabetic random	< 99	Diabetes is unlikely
Non diabetic fasting	99-138	Further investigation is required and needs a clinical referral
Non diabetic random	138-150	Further investigation is required and refer to the doctor
Diabetic	> 180	Needs medical attention

Individuals who could benefit from the screening of blood glucose include

- Patients who are expressing anxiety about the development of diabetes mellitus
- Whose diabetes was controlled by diet alone or by oral hypoglycemic drugs.
- Individuals who are diabetic and require regular blood glucose monitoring for evaluating the drug therapy.

- Individuals showing symptoms of diabetes such as poly urea, poly phasia, tiredness and weight loss etc.,

Appropriate measurement of capillary blood glucose is useful to detect the fresh cases of diabetes mellitus. Capillary blood glucose can be measured by using glucometer which is a small electronic device. Following are the normal values of capillary blood glucose.

CBG	Capillary Blood Glucose Value
Fasting CBG	70 – 100 mg/dl
Post Prandial CBG	110 – 150 mg/dl
Random CBG	100 – 150 mg/dl

Techniques for measurement of blood glucose by glucometer:

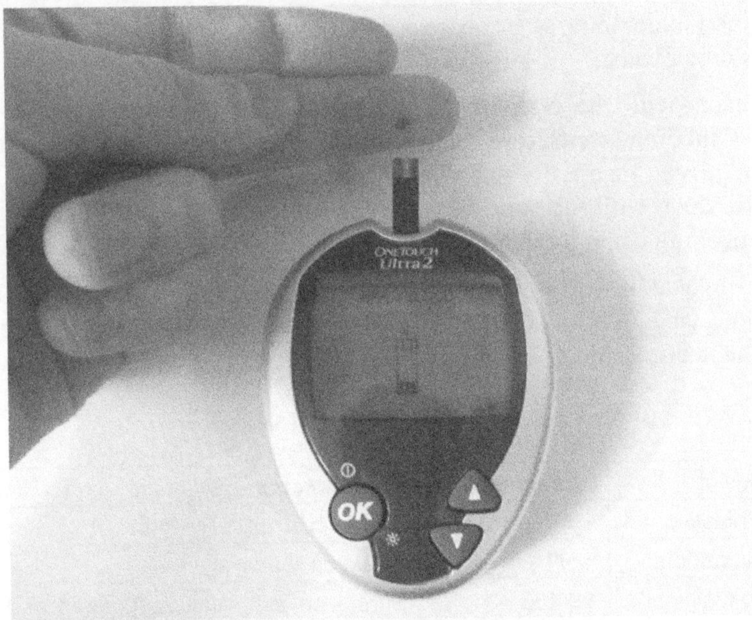

Fig. 6.2 Measuring Blood Glucose

- A blood glucose test is performed by piercing the skin (typically, on the finger sterilized using alcohol cotton swab) applying a small drop of blood on to a chemically active disposable 'test-strip' which the digital meter calorimetrically detects and read. Within 5 seconds, the capillary blood glucose value will be displayed on the glucometer screen (Fig. 6.2)
- The fasting capillary blood glucose level (FBG), capillary random blood sugar (RBS) and capillary postprandial blood sugar (PPBS) can be measured using glucometer.
- The values of capillary blood glucose measured should be provided in verbal and written form to consult a physician if there is high blood glucose level.

CALCULATION OF BODY MASS INDEX (BMI)

Body Mass Index (BMI) is a statistical measure of body fat based on height and weight that applies to both adult men and women. BMI is the most widely used diagnostic tool to identify weight problems whether individuals are underweight, overweight or obese. Following are the formulas used to calculate BMI.

Formula to calculate the BMI

BMI = Weight (kg)/Height (m) x Height (m)

English BMI formula

BMI= (weight in pounds/(Height in inches) x (Height in inches)] x 703

Categorization based on BMI

Category	BMI range – kg/m^2
Severely underweight	less than 16.5
Under weight	from 16.5 to 18.4
Normal	from 18.5 to 24.9
Overweight	from 25 to 30
Obese Class I	from 30.1 to 34.9
Obese Class II	from 35 to 40
Obese Class III	over 40

MEASUREMENT OF PEAK EXPIRATORY FLOW RATE (PEFR)

During Asthma and Chronic Obstructive Pulmnary Disease (COPD), patients will have decreased airway ventilation due to bronchoconstriction. In such situations, Peak Expiratory Flow Rate (PEFR) is a useful device to assess the lung function in such patients. This test also helps patient and pharmacist in identifying the usefulness of bronchodilators in the management of asthma or COPD. Peak flow meter is a small device used to measure the person's maximum speed of expiration. PEFR readings are useful in determining the lung functionality, severity of asthma symptoms and treatment options.

Techniques for measurement of peak expiratory flow rate (PEFR) by peak flow meter:

- Check to place the peak flow meter pointer at zero
- Preferably make the patient stand or sit in a comfortable, upright position
- Hold the peak flow meter level (horizontally) and keep the fingers away from the pointer
- Ask the patient to take a deep breath and close lips firmly around the mouthpiece
- Then ask the patient to blow as hard as possible
- Look at the pointer and check the reading (Fig. 6.3).

- Reset the pointer back to zero and do this three times and record the highest reading
- The higher PEFR values indicates patients are well and lower PEFR values indicates airways are constricted
- The PEFR 80-100% indicates that the person is relatively symptom free; PEFR 50-80% indicates caution should be taken and condition is worsening, and PEFR below 50% indicates that the disease is in a very severe condition.

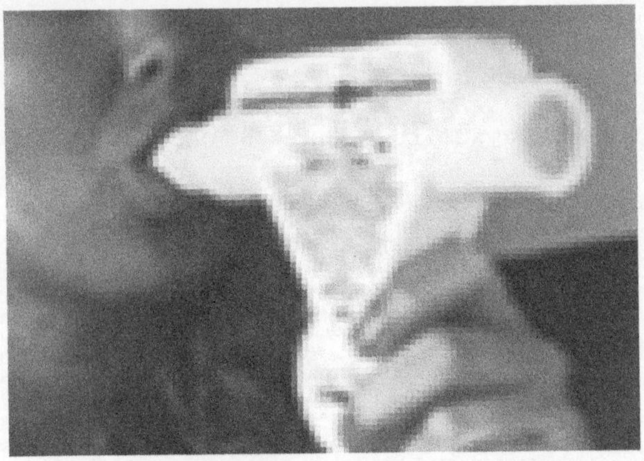

Fig. 6.3 Measuring PEFR

KEY POINTS

- Health screening services in community pharmacies helps in identifying the newly developed hypertensive and diabetic patients.
- Health screening services by community pharmacists will improve the pharmaceutical care process and also helps in improving the professional relationship with both patient and the doctor.
- For providing health screening services, the pharmacist should take adequate training and follow the correct procedures to give the result.

SUGGESTED READINGS

1. Screening for Type 2 Diabetes Report of a World Health Organization and International Diabetes Federation meeting 2003.
2. Shane Jackson and Gregory Peterson (2006). Health screening services: an update. *Australian Pharmacist* **25(11):** 846-851.
3. UK National Screening Committee. Criteria for appraising the viability, effectiveness and appropriateness of a screening programme 2009. Last accessed April 22, 2009.

CHAPTER 7

MEDICATION ADHERENCE

LEARNING OBJECTIVES

- Define medication adherence
- Understand the factors responsible for medication nonadherence
- Know the role of the pharmacist in improving medication adherence

Drugs do not work if patients' do not take them

-Everett C Koop, M.D

In patient care, the next important step after the correct diagnosis is giving the prescriptions to patients to manage their disease conditions. Although any amount of care is taken for diagnosis, the success of the therapy takes place only when patients take their medicines as their doctor advised. World Health Organisation defines medication adherence as **"the extent to which a person's behavior in taking medications corresponds with the agreed recommendations from a health care provider".**

The word compliance and adherence are not synonyms. Compliance is often confused as adherence. Compliance suggests that patient is passively following the doctor's order with out any established professional relationship. Where as in medication adherence, doctor and patient discuss the therapeutic plan such as drug dosing time, how to take the medicine etc., and work on the opportunities to improve the adherence to the medication.

In recent times, the word **"concordance"** is used, which is more realistic and is based on the patient and the prescriber's relationship.

Numerous research studies have shown that, adherence to medication decreases the illness, disability, and death. Despite of such findings, people often do not take the medications regularly.

TYPES OF MEDICATION NON-ADHERENCE

Normally patients tend to miss the medication dose due to various reasons is termed as medication non-adherence. Missing the administration of medication doses may be willful or unintentional. Further medication non-adherence is classified as

1. Primary non-adherence
2. Secondary non-adherence

1. **Primary non-adherence to medication:** If a patient fails to get his/her prescription dispensed is called as primary non-adherence to medication.
2. **Secondary non-adherence to medication:** Secondary non-adherence to medication is further classified as

   (a) Intentional non-adherence (b) Unintentional non-adherence

   (a) ***Intentional non-adherence to medication:*** Intentional non-adherence to medication is defined as if patient willfully deviate the instructions given by the doctor such as taking fewer doses than the prescribed or taking more doses than the prescribed in anticipation of increased benefit or discontinuation of medication prematurely when the symptoms were decreased or disappeared, or taking the medication with prohibited foods, liquids, and other medications, and improper use of medication administration devices.

   (b) ***Unintentional non-adherence to medication:*** Unintentional non-adherence results mainly when a patient misunderstood the instructions given by the doctor or forgotten to take medicines as advised due to cognitive problems.

Medication non-adherence is also classified based on the extent of medication use by the patients as

(i) Adherent (ii) Partially adherent (iii) Non-adherent

(i) **Adherent:** A person is called as adherent to the medication when he or she takes the medication more than 80% of the prescribed doses.

(ii) **Partially adherent:** A person is termed as partially adherent when he or she takes the medication between 70-80% of the prescribed doses.

(iii) **Non-adherent:** A person is called as non adherent to the medication when he or she takes the medication less than 70% of the prescribed doses.

INTELLIGENT NON ADHERENCE

Intelligent non adherence was first coined by Weintraub. Intelligent non adherence means if a person willfully stops medication due to some adverse effects such as nausea, vomiting or gastric irritation etc., by cessation of the medication, if the condition improves then it is called as intelligent non adherence.

Clinical Situations Requiring Medication Adherence

Following are the clinical situations which demands high rate of adherence to the medication.

1. Maintenance of body metabolic activity: E.g., Insulin and Thyroxin deficiency disorders.
2. Chronic disease conditions like Hypertension and Diabetes to prevent complications.

3. Ailments that require a uniform plasma concentration of the medication. E.g., Epilepsy
4. Chronic infections having public interest like Tuberculosis, Hepatitis and HIV.

Medication adherence research studies opine that for achieving the desired therapeutic goals, more than 90% medication adherence is essential. In case of HIV infection, research has demonstrated that suboptimal adherence (i.e., taking less than 90-95% of prescribed doses) is associated with increased risk of adverse virologic and clinical outcomes, including increased viral replication and the development of drug-resistant HIV strains.

In hypertensive patients, adherence to antihypertensive is essential. A Meta analysis of the research findings of 61 studies has observed the less incidences of ischemic heart diseases and stroke deaths in individuals who maintained more than 90% of medication adherence.

Consequences of Medication Non-adherence

Non-adherence to the medications has a great influence on patient and the health care system. Research studies have shown that the non adherence to the medications is associated with

(a) Poorer health outcomes
(b) Increased utilization of health care resources
(c) High health care expenditures

This is particularly evident in case of chronic disorders like hypertension, ischemic heart disease, diabetes and asthma. Inadequate medication adherence may lead to treatment failures and recurrence of the disease. Tuberculosis is caused by *Mycobacterium Tuberculosis* a leading communicable disease and considered as one of the top ten diseases contributing for global mortality. The most serious problem hindering the control of tuberculosis is non adherence of patients to the antitubercular medications. This delays the conversion of sputum positive to smear negative, increase the relapse rates by 5 - 6 times, and produces the resistant mutant strains.

Medication non-adherence is also associated with deceased quality of life. Some interventional studies have demonstrated the increased quality of life in patients who were adherent to their medications.

Factors Affecting the Medication Adherence

World Health Organisation (WHO) has termed medication adherence as multi dimensional phenomena and classified the factors affecting medication adherence in to the following classes.

1. Social and economic factors
2. Health care system factors
3. Condition related factors

4. Therapy related factors
5. Patient related factors

1. **Social and economic factors:** Social and economic factors for non-adherence to medication include people with low health literacy, without family or social support network, unstable living conditions (homelessness), busy schedules at office or at the business, limited access to health care facilities, inability or difficulty of access to the pharmacy, high cost of medications, cultural and lay benefits about illness and treatment
2. **Health care system factors:** Factors under the health care system contributing to medication non-adherence includes poor relationship between the provider and the patient, poor communication of the provider, disparity between health belief models of the provider and the patient. Inadequate reinforcement by the health care provider, lack of a system to educate both provider and the patients about the disease, and its appropriate management, and lack of continuity of care also are the contributing factors for medication non-adherence.
3. **Condition related factors:** Condition related factors include decrease in symptom severity, or disappearance of the symptoms, patients with depression may not show interest to take medications, and patients with psychiatric disorders do not remember to take the medications.
4. **Therapy related factors:** Complexity of the therapeutic regimen, treatment requiring mastery of techniques (injections and inhalers), duration of therapy, frequent changes in the medication regimen, lack of immediate benefit of therapy, medication use attached with social stigma, unpleasant side effects, and treatment interference with life style or requires significant behavioral changes.
5. **Patient related factors:** Patient related factors include visual impairment, hearing impairment, cognitive impairment, impaired mobility or dexterity, swallowing problems, poor understanding about the disease and benefits of medication usage, inadequate motivation from health care providers or family members, fear of adverse effects, psychosocial stress, anxiety or anger.

Formula to Calculate Medication Adherence

%Adherence =

$$\frac{\text{Total number of actual doses the patient has consumed since last appointment}}{\text{Total number of calculated doses to be consumed}} \; 100$$

Role of Pharmacist in Improving the Medication Adherence

Pharmacist can work with patients in removing the health system related factors. One of the major barriers for patients' non-adherence to their medications is lack of belief about the useful role of medications in the management of disease. In most of the situations, doctors only give prescriptions than having dialogue with patient about the medications and their usage and strategies to incorporate the regimen in to the daily routine. Patients are also worried about the adverse effects associated with the medications which they were prescribed.

Many research studies have confirmed that, pharmacist can play an important role in improving the medication adherence behavior through patient counseling. During the counseling, pharmacist can identify the factors responsible for non adherence to medication in the patient and through discussion pharmacist can change the attitude of the patient and can motivate them to improve the medication adherence behavior.

KEY POINTS

- Treatment outcomes are directly influenced by patients' adherence behavior to their medication.
- Social and economic factors, health care system factors, therapy related factors, patient related factors influences the patient's medication adherence behavior.
- Pharmacist can play very important role in improving the medication adherence behavior.

SUGGESTED READINGS

1. Ines. K, Susan J. Taylor, Carlene Smith, Carol L. Armour. Impact on Medication Use and Adherence of Australian Pharmacists: Diabetes Care Services. J AmPharm Assoc 2005; **45:** 33-40.
2. John A Gans (2003). Improving Medication Adhernce: Pharmacists should take the Lead. *Journal of the American Pharmacists* **43(6):** 665.
3. Medication adherence in America. A National report. http://www.ncpanet.org/pdf/reportcard/AdherenceReportCard_Full.pdf
4. Medication Adherence Time Tool: Improving Health Outcomes- A Resource from the American College of Preventive Medicine. http://www.acpm.org/?MedAdherTT_ClinRef
5. Phillippe Sudre, Stephane Jacquemet, Christophe Uldry, Thomas V Perneger (1999). Objectives, methods and content of patient education programmes for adults with asthma: Systemic review of studies published between 1979 and 1998. Thorax; **54:** 681-687.

CHAPTER **8**

COMMUNITY PHARMACY MANAGEMENT

LEARNING OBJECTIVES

- Know the legal requirements to start a community pharmacy.
- Understand the importance of site selection.
- Appreciate various designs of the pharmacy and layout.
- Know and maintain various registers in the pharmacy.

INTRODUCTION

In the last census, India had crossed one billion population with an exponential addition of 30 million population every year. Due to overcrowded population, poor sanitation, limited medical facilities people are suffering from various diseases such as infectious diseases like Malaria, Filaria, Tuberculosis, Leprosy, Cholera and Gastroenteritis, Helminthic infestation, Polio, AIDS and other Sexually Transmitted Diseases. Malnutrition disorders include anemia, and vitamin deficiency diseases are in high rise. Since Independence, although the governments are introducing many health care programs for improving the public health maternal and infant deaths are not under control. In urban and semi urban areas the problems are different. Social habits such as cigarette smoking, chewing pan masala and gutka and alcohol consumption are increasing and leading to many diseases like asthma, chronic obstructive pulmonary disorders (COPD), hypertension, diabetes, gastro intestinal and liver diseases. Most of the people in the productive age group are becoming slaves for these social habits and becoming burden to the society. In communities when people become sick, they will first visit the nearby medical store for receiving the primary care. If symptoms do not resolve, than patients will go to the clinics for consulting the doctor.

In India, people often call community pharmacies as Medical stores, Medical shop, Medical and General Stores. Community pharmacists are suitably qualified and are in the right position to help such people by providing the right medication for right patient with suitable advice for medication usage, conducting awareness camps, group counseling and smoking cessation programs and other health care programs. The Community Pharmacy is defined as "a place where the medicines are stocked and dispensed to the patients or patient care givers under the supervision of a qualified and registered pharmacist upon the production of a prescription or when legally permitted without the prescription". Community Pharmacy is not only a place for professional services but it is also a business establishment. Success of a community pharmacy depends upon various important aspects such as location of the pharmacy, design of the pharmacy, display of the goods, approach of the pharmacy personnel, and provision of patient care services.

Site Selection

Although community pharmacy practice is a profession but predominantly it is a trade. So apart from providing the services, it is essential to take suitable steps to improve the business. Before starting the pharmacy, the pharmacist should do a macro survey of the area where he or she is intending to start the business such as the population size, number of practicing doctors, number of medical stores existing around should be taken in to the consideration. Suitable selection of the site is very important for a good business. A site chosen correctly can boom the business and a wrongly chosen site may run the business in to losses since the pharmacy business depends upon the prescription feed. The prescription feed come from attached doctor or nearby practicing doctor or nearby hospital, or floating prescriptions. To receive the prescriptions from all the possible sources, it is essential to open the pharmacy which is close by to prescription feed sources. The suitable sites for opening a pharmacy are

(a) Attached to a clinic
(b) Close by to clinics
(c) Nearby to a hospital
(d) In a busy market
(e) Growing city extensions
(f) Close by to railway station or bus station

(a) ***Attached to a clinic:*** This is the most suitable site for opening a pharmacy. The prescriber will send you a very good number of prescriptions based on your rapport with him and the service you give to your clients. The advantages of this kind of the set up is regular prescription feed, substitution may be permitted when the prescribed brand is not available at that moment. Patients may also consider the pharmacist as first of contact for health related information and advice.

(b) ***Close by to clinics:*** It is also considered as a good choice to open a pharmacy close by to the clinics in a colony or in a market area. Advantages of opening the pharmacy in such areas is good prescription feed from the general practitioners, permission for substitution when prescribed brand is not available, good customer rapport and opportunity for general OTC sales. The pharmacist in co-operation and taking the confidence of the doctor can provide pharmaceutical care services such as counseling, drug therapy management through health screening services. These services will improve the patient confidence about the pharmacist as health care professional and contribute for the success of the business.

(c) *Nearly to hospital:* Opening a pharmacy nearby to a government general hospital or any other secondary care or tertiary care hospital is a good idea. The opportunity for prescription feed will be high. However the pharmacist requires maintaining wide variety of product range with different brands. If appropriate inventories are maintained, this is a good option for successful business. The disadvantages are less rapport with the prescribing doctor and poor chances of brand substitution, maintaining more number of brands will influence the inventory costs.

(d) *In a busy market:* Busy markets are also considered as right choices for opening the pharmacies due to increased movement of the public in these areas. Public may visit the market for purchasing different commodities. Along with purchase of other commodities, they will also tend to purchase the medicines for their health care. The pharmacies opened in busy markets will primarily depend on the floating prescriptions. Success of such pharmacy depends upon layout and design of the pharmacy with patient waiting area, water facilities, patient care services such as counseling, health screening services, and cash discount. On long run, customer patronage will increase the business volume, which in turn increases the profit margin. Shopping malls, close by cinema theaters are also other good options to open the pharmacies.

(e) *Growing city extensions:* Growing city extensions are also good sites for opening community pharmacies. People in such areas find difficulty in going to market for emergency requirement of medicines. If a pharmacy is opened with facilities such as patient waiting area, counseling and health screening services area will attract the customers. Chronic patients like diabetes, asthma may require detailed counseling on safe and effective use of insulin injections or inhalers. If such facilities are provided patients will be pleased to patronize the pharmacies. The pharmacist can also make the pharmacy popularize in the area by conducting health promotion programs and health camps etc. This type of pharmacies will have good opportunities for pharmaceutical care services.

(f) *Close by to railway station or bus station:* Railway stations and bus stations are also considered as good locations for opening the pharmacies. The commuters may require medicines to get an immediate relief for acute conditions such as diarrhea, common colds, or body aches. Availability of a pharmacy in close by to these areas will help the patients to purchase the medicines. This type of pharmacies will receive the floating prescriptions and prescriptions for acute conditions. Along with prescription medicines, opportunity for generic sales will be also very high in contributing to the business volume.

Apart from the above, other important criteria required to be considered by the pharmacists while opening a pharmacy are

(a) Parking space in front of the pharmacy
(b) Close by Traffic lights and traffic rules
(c) Visibility of the pharmacy
(d) Expansion opportunity for the existing space

(e) Clear negotiations with the land lord regarding the rent or lease of the pharmacy
(f) Facilities for temperature control for thermo labile medicines
(g) Separate storage spaces for poison and Schedule X drugs

SPACE LAYOUT AND DESIGN

In the modern world the clients will always give importance for quality services in short possible time. Especially in service oriented establishments, preference also will be given for interiors and ambience. To meet this demand it is essential to have a new work system and facility design for the community pharmacies. The new work system should be developed to optimize the utilization of space, and sales personnel time and allow the pharmacist to increase patient care services without adding the personnel. In the new design, pharmacists should be able to review prescriptions, check technicians' work, and dispense prescriptions, counseling patients as needed; technicians would enter prescriptions into the pharmacy computer and fill them.

The objectives of a good pharmacy layout is to

- Attract maximum number of customers
- Provide an opportunity for the customers to purchase more
- Create a pleasant ambiance in the pharmacy and provide basic amenities for the clients with maximum space utilization
- Provide customer convenience and the satisfaction
- Minimize the salary expenses through layout efficiency and space utilization.

Based on the layout and design, the pharmacies can be classified as

(a) Prescription oriented traditional pharmacy design
(b) Super drug store pharmacy design
(c) Pharmacy with pharmaceutical care services design

PRESCRIPTION ORIENTED TRADITIONAL PHARMACY DESIGN

These are the traditional drug stores which are commonly seen in the market or street side. Major objective of such pharmacies is to serve the customers through filling maximum number of prescriptions and sale of other products to increase the business volume. In such pharmacies, the lay out will include a cash counter with facilities for billing and collection of the cash. The product display will be in racks supported with the sales man service. Customer choice and selection will be very limited. Amenities for customers are also very limited. Dimensions of such pharmacies will be around 200 Sq.ft

Model layout of the Traditional Pharmacy Design

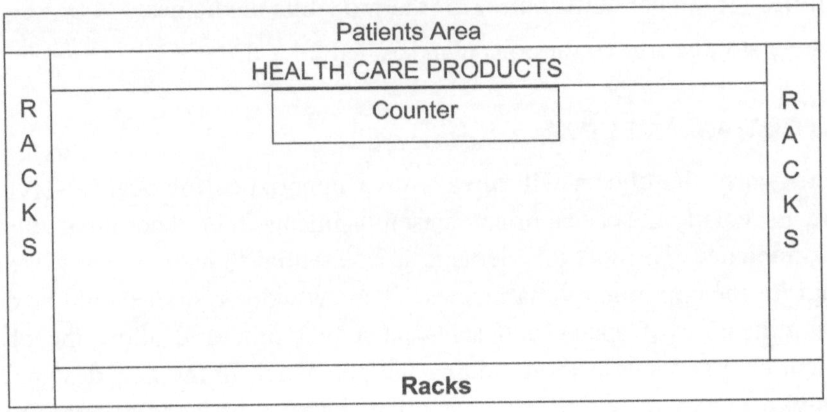

SUPER DRUG STORE PHARMACY DESIGN

Super drug store pharmacy designs are more common in the western world. These pharmacies will provide opportunity for purchase of both prescription and other general health care items, cosmetics, baby care, eye care and other gift items. In such pharmacies, along with separate prescription counter, sales man supported health care items counter, gift items counter will be present. The pharmacy should also have a separate attached place to collect the goods and storage before the goods are displayed. The ambience and design of the pharmacy are made in such a way to attract more customers with increased purchasing temptation. Along with prescription items, sales for general items also will contribute for the business volume.

Model Layout of Superdrug Store Pharmacy Designs

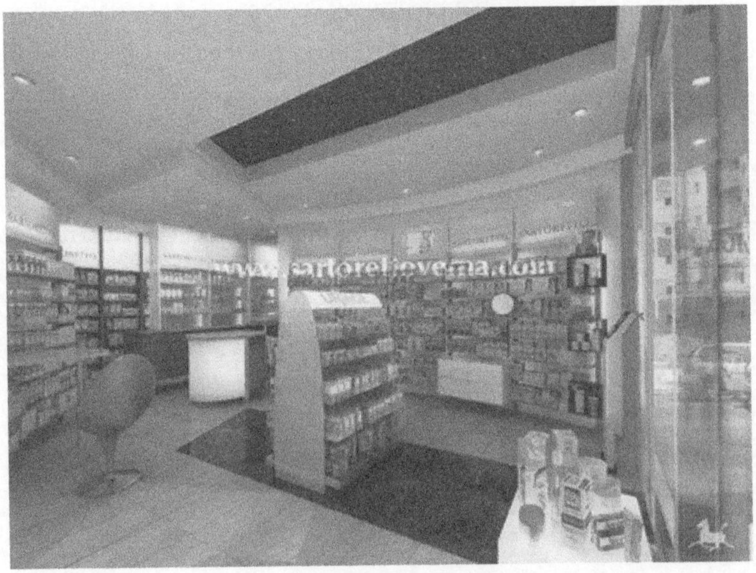

PHARMACY WITH PHARMACEUTICAL CARE SERVICES DESIGN

Pharmaceutical care is a responsible provision of drug therapy to achieve the desired therapeutic goals. Pharmacies with pharmaceutical care services will have separate patient care area for offering counseling and health screening services along with area for display of medicines and other health care items supported with sales man service. The design should include space for prescription counter, a separate counter for other health care items, toiletries, and baby care items display and sales. The wrapping and billing counter should be at the entrance.

Optimum Design Characteristics of a Pharmacy

- The pharmacy should be painted with special light professional colors to give a serene and pleasant feeling to the customers when they enter the pharmacy.
- The pharmacy should be well illuminated with proper ventilation or air conditioned and with appealing room freshener.
- Basic amenities such as customer waiting area with seating facility, availability of health magazines for reading while the prescriptions are filled, with wash room facility should be created. Water and espresso coffee facility may add value to the customer care.
- A separate counter should be made available for prescription medicines with pharmacist services.
- A separate pharmaceutical care service for patient care, special counseling cubicle with health screening service equipment.
- Display of health care items, toiletries and gifts should in a separate corner with sales person assisted services.
- Adequate fixtures and furniture should be made in the design of pharmacy for stocking all varieties of medicines.

Legal Requirements to Start a Community Pharmacy

In order to sell drugs and pharmaceuticals, the pharmacy should comply with all the provisions of the Drugs and Cosmetics Act 1940. Any individual to open a pharmacy to sell medicines in retail or wholesale or sale of drugs by retail without engaging service of a qualified person (restricted licence), sale of drugs by wholesale from a Motor Vehicle, sale of homeopathic medicines by wholesale or retail should obtain the prescribed licence from the licensing authority. For obtaining licence to sell drugs in above categories, following application forms may be used.

List of Application Forms, Licenses Categories of Drugs to Be Sold

S. No.	Appl. Form Number	Category of Drugs to be sold	Presence of qualified person required	Form Number in which licence is issued for categories of drugs
1	19	Wholesale/Retail of drugs other than specified in Schedule X	Yes	20- For retail sale of Category A drugs 20 B Wholesale of category A drugs 21 - Sale of category B drugs 21 B wholesale of category B drugs 21 C renewal of licenses 20 A & B and 21 A & B
2	19 A	Restricted Licence	No	20 A- retail sales of category A drugs and 21 A- retail sale of category B drugs.
3	19 AA	Sale of drugs from Motor Vehicle	Yes	20 BB wholesale of category A drugs 21 BB wholesale of category B drugs
4	19 B	Wholesale/Retail sale of Homeopathic medicines	Yes	20 C- Sale by retail 20 D- Sale by wholesale 20 E - Renewal of License – 20 C/20 D
5	19 C	Wholesale/Retail sale of drugs specified in Schedule X	Yes	20 F sale by retail 20 G sale by wholesale 20 C Renewal of above

Procedure to Obtain the Licence

An applicant to sell the drugs of A category, B Category and Schedule X drugs in retail should apply to the Drugs Control Department in a suitable application form with the prescribed fee. Along with the application form, the following documents are required to be attached.

(a) The layout of the premises, where pharmacy is going to be started (The minimum area required to start a retail pharmacy is 120 Sqft.)

(b) The rent agreement between the landlord and the applicant

(c) Invoice proof of purchase of the refrigerator for stocking the Schedule C & C_1 drugs.

(d) The in-charge person should be a qualified person who is a registered pharmacist.

For granting the licence, the licensing authority will inspect the premises and upon satisfaction will issue the license to start the pharmacy.

Staff

Pharmacy business is not only trade but also a profession. As per the Drugs and Cosmetics Act, all the medicines should be dispensed under the supervision of a qualified person. In Indian context, a person passed 2 year Diploma in Pharmacy (D. Pharm) and undergone practical training of 500 hours in a hospital pharmacy or community pharmacy or a B. Pharm graduate with 150 hours of practical training is also eligible to register in State Pharmacy Council as a pharmacist. Only such registered pharmacists are called as qualified persons. To assist the qualified persons in pharmacy operations, individuals with other qualifications such as 10+2 qualification or degree may be appointed as pharmacy assistants. The patient focused pharmacy program Pharm D was started in 2008 by Pharmacy Council of India. Pharm D graduates are trained to take the responsibility in managing the overall activities of pharmacy including patient focused services such as patient counseling, health screening services and drug therapy monitoring. Pharm D graduates will really add value to the pharmacy through patient care services.

Materials-Coding, Stocking

When medicines are received from the supplier i.e., wholesaler, the stocks should be properly arranged in the racks for easy location and removal of the drug from its carton box at the time of dispensing. Various methods are adopted by the pharmacists as per their choice and convenience. Such as company wise, product wise or pharmacological category wise etc., the methods used for coding the stocks are classified in to:

(a) Mnemonic method
(b) Scientific method
(c) Random method

(a) ***Mnemonic method:*** Mnemonic means "memory". In order to remember easily the location of particular category of medicines, a suitable code may be used such as "GI" for all the categories of drugs that are used to treat Gastro Intestinal disorders. On the top of the medicine cabinet, a label can be fixed stating "GI".

(b) ***Scientific method:*** In the scientific method, all medicines may be divided into various categories such as therapeutic classification. This may be further subdivided into dosage forms. A simple example of this is major therapeutic class is "Cardiovascular Drugs" The drugs under this class may be further sub divided in to HTN, which mean the drugs used to treat hypertension. Further all the drugs used to treat hypertension such as Diuretics, Beta Blockers, Calcium Channel Blockers, Angiotensin Convertase Enzyme Inhibitors (ACEI) or Angiotensin Receptor Blockers (ARB) may be further coded as DU, BB, CCB, ACEI and ARB. Based on the type of dosage form, the medicines may also be coded.

(c) ***Random method:*** It is more like an arbitrary method. Medicines may be stored in alphabetical order or in numeral order or dosage form order.

Various health care items are sold in the pharmacy such as prescription medicines, OTC medicines and other health care and surgical items. It is very difficult to remember the location of the items before they are sold. Thus in order to remember their location, location coding also may adopted keeping the type of item, supplier wise or company wise.

All medicines received from the stockiest should be taken in to the central store. From there the stocks may be taken in to the pharmacy in small quantities where they may be dispensed. This act will help the retailer in assessing inventory needs.

Maintenance of Various Registers in the Pharmacy

For the successful operation of the pharmacy activities, following registers should be maintained.

(a) Inventory registers

(b) Cash register

(c) Ledger

USE OF COMPUTERS: BUSINESS AND HEALTH CARE SOFT WARES

In recent times, computers have become a very important tool in all areas of science and technology. With the proliferation of the internet and the developments in computer technology, number of computer applications is increased. In the field of pharmacy, computers are used starting from drug designing & development to patient care. Various hardware and software have been developed to meet the needs of pharmaceutical industry and hospital & community pharmacy. Further development is still in progress which will make pharmacist's job easier. Following are the applications of computers in community pharmacy.

1. Communication
2. Prescription Processing
3. Checking the pharmaceutical care
4. Inventory control
5. Accountancy

1. *Communication:* Computers are used within pharmacies to facilitate communication. From email to other internet-based messaging systems, online communication allows pharmacists and other pharmacy staff to keep in contact both within their own organization and also within the professional community. Some pharmacy chain companies have their own intranet systems for internal communications over the Internet.
2. *Prescription processing:* Prescription processing is invariably one of the main activities going on within a pharmacy on a day-to-day basis, and computers are used to make this process more reliable and efficient. Both the customer service side of pharmacy operation and the dispensing aspects are today carried out through the use

of computing systems. Pharmacy computers also handle customer service activities such as sales and cash handling within the retail operation.

3. ***Error prevention:*** Pharmacy computer systems can help to prevent errors in prescriptions, potentially saving lives and generally preserving the health of patients. As well as checking medicines and combinations of medicines, these systems can in some cases check on patient information. Availability of such systems varies across the different geographical areas, but in some cases pharmacy computers are able to check on prescribed medicines with specific reference to a patient and their overall health-care picture.
4. ***Inventory control:*** Pharmacy software is so designed to give the accurate stock position at any point of time and also to give reorder levels.
5. ***Accountancy:*** Community pharmacy is a retail business where all transactions are of financial nature. Thus it is very essential to record, classify and summarize all the financial transactions in order to know the profit and loss in the business. Thus accounting system is mandatory in any business. Accounting is defined "as the process of identifying, measuring and communicating economic information in a business".

Accounting is a guide post for investors for investing into the business, for creditors to advance money to the firm and to the government to know its functioning and to consumers for price changes.

SYSTEMS OF ACCOUNTING

Following are the main systems available to record all the business transactions.

(a) Cash system

(b) Mercantile system

(c) Mixed system

(a) ***Cash system:*** In cash system actual receipts and payments of cash transactions are recorded. This system does not help in knowing the exact financial position of the business at a particular day.

(b) ***Mercantile system:*** Under this system all transactions relating to a period is recorded in the books of accounts including the income receivable and payable. This system gives a complete picture of financial transactions of the business and discloses correct profit or loss and exhibits true financial position of the business on a particular day.

(c) ***Mixed system:*** Under this system both cash system and mercantile systems are used. Some transactions are kept under cash system and others are under mercantile system.

Accounting Cycle

An accounting cycle includes the following steps:

(a) Recording all business transactions in to a primary book called as journal or in its subsidiary books.

(b) Posting of transactions in to the ledger.

(c) Preparation of final accounts.

At the end of the financial year final accounts may be prepared following the accounting cycle and this continues for whole life of the business.

Objectives of Accountancy

Accountancy helps us to

1. Know the profit and loss of business during a particular period.
2. Understand the financial position of the business such as assets and liabilities.
3. Know the progress of the business.
4. Comply with the legal requirements.

HUMAN RELATIONS AND COMMUNICATIONS

Concept of pharmacy practice has changed from product focus to patient focused in recent years. The pharmacy profession has undergone an extensive self analysis and reevaluation of its duties and objectives. The result of reexamination has focused more emphasis on incorporation of clinical pharmacy in patient care. It is now universally recognized that pharmacist is far more than a mere dispenser of the drugs but is pharmaceutical care provider. The pharmacist has the following important duties:

(a) It is important to analyze the medication's safety from patients' past medication and medical history.

(b) To identify any known allergies, drug interactions or other contraindications in a given prescription.

(c) To ensure that patients uses their medicines appropriately as indicated.

Pharmacy operations are not just mere billing the medications and distributing to the patients. An element of personal care by the pharmacist improves the customer satisfaction and increases the patronage of the client to the pharmacy.

Attitude and Appearance

Attitude is the overall emotional stance of an individual towards his/her job responsibilities, clients, employers, and other colleagues. Appearance is the overall look of an employee during his job including the dress and grooming. It is expected that the pharmacist should look like a professional by wearing a formal dress with an apron and a name tag, greeting the customers with smile and make the eye contact while talking to them. Respond politely to customer with their queries, and at the same time respect their privacy. Use of common courteous words in every interaction such as "Good Morning", "Have a nice day", "Please", and "Thank You" should become a part of their regular vocabulary. Pharmacist should be sensitive to cultural and language differences. If the pharmacist cannot understand a customer because of the language difference, it is better to apologize for the language deficiency and take the help of other employee or other store employee to translate the conversation. Cultural differences also should be taken in to account. If the pharmacy is located in an area, where people of particular community reside, try to understand their diet, health habits or beliefs and courtesies. Knowing more about the culture will help us to understand them and provide services in better way and this will satisfy the clients.

KEY POINTS

- Community pharmacy is a first point of contact for public to get the treatment for minor ailments and to receive the prescription medicines.
- To have good customer patronage, it is essential to open the pharmacy where public movement or patients' movement is high.
- Good location and attractive ambience with patient care facilities increases the customer patronage.
- Pharmacists should know the legal requirements to open the pharmacy and accordingly all licenses should be obtained from the regulatory authorities.
- Pharmacists with professional attire and with good communication skills make a positive impact on patients.

SUGGESTED READINGS

1. Mohammed Ali and Jyoti Gupta. Drug Store and Business management. CBS Publishers and Distributors, New Delhi.
2. Mohan Singhal and Jai Dev. Drug Store and Business Management. Vikas & Co. Jalandar.
3. S H Merchant, J.S. Quadry. A text book of retail pharmacy management. B.S.Shah Prakashan, Ahmedabad.

CHAPTER 9

INVENTORY CONTROL IN COMMUNITY PHARMACY

LEARNING OBJECTIVES

- Define inventory control.
- Know the objectives of inventory control.
- Understand the different methods of inventory control.

INTRODUCTION

In community pharmacies, pharmacists procure medicines from licensed authorized wholesalers or distributors and stock them adequately and dispense. The whole activity looks very simple and straightforward. However an effective procurement process ensures the availability of all the medicines in the right quantities at reasonable prices at all the times. This will ensure better cash rotation, excellent customer service, and improved professional relationship with the suppliers, fair returns on investments, and future growth of the business. Thus it is very important to understand the art of inventory control of medicines in the pharmacy in order to avoid "out of stock" and "over stock" situations. These situations will result in loss of clientele and future business. An effective inventory control practices helps the pharmacist to avoid these embarrassing situations.

Inventory control is defined as "the supervision of procurement, storage and accessibility of items in order to ensure an adequate supply of medicines in right time". Inventory control is also defined as the itemized list of medicines procured in the right quantity, right quality, at right time in the right price from the right suppliers. Procurement of medicines from the suppliers depends upon the sales/demand of a particular medicine and the decision of the pharmacist/person in charge of ordering, discounts received from the manufacturer and wholesaler. Thus credit and inventory control requires knowledge and skill in assessing the market demand, period of discount, distance between the wholesaler and retailer, supply policies of wholesaler, buying capacity, and transport facilities. Thus inventory control is an art and science.

Procurement of stocks and managing the inventory is an important function of the pharmacy and part of Good Pharmacy Practice. Inefficient procurements negatively impact the profits of the pharmacy. Pharmacists can prepare and implement standard guidelines/systems and written procedures, regarding smooth procurement and inventory management. Procurement involves the selection of medicines, assessing the quantity required, assessing the availability of sufficient funds, selecting the suppliers, obtaining the best deals and services, placing the orders, verifying the stocks ordered and actual stocks received, taking them into the stocks, making the payments to the suppliers.

STEPS FOR INVENTORY CONTROL

Effective Procurement

Effective procurement begins from reviewing the customers' requirements market need. This includes the need of the prescribers, patients, patrons and other general population. Few factors such as location of the pharmacy, clientele, pharmacy image, specialized services the pharmacy offers will also influence the procurement practices. The cycle of procurement is depicted in the below flow chart.

Flow chart of effective procurement

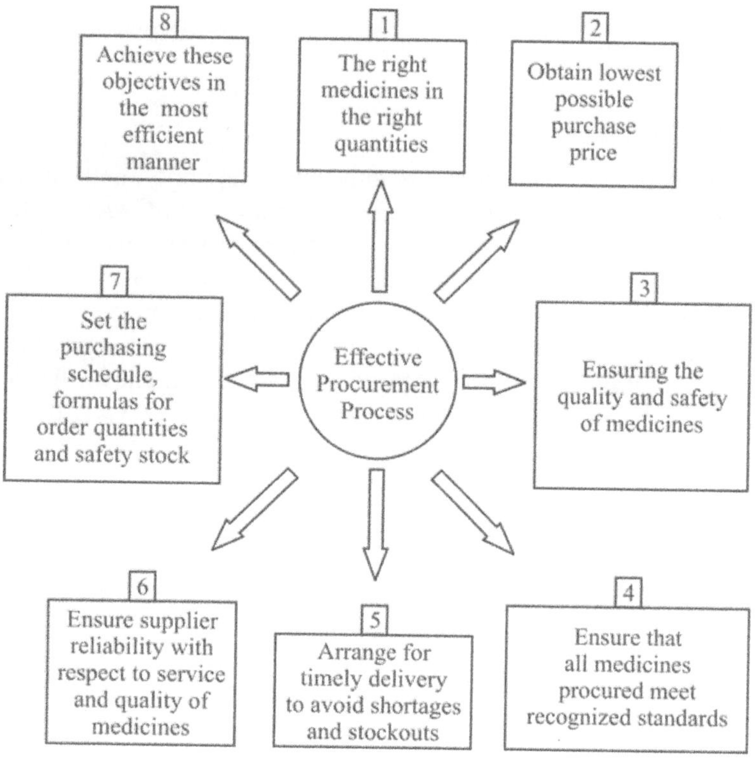

Selection of the Medicines

Accurate estimate for selection of medicines is important to avoid stock out and overstock of medicines. In India currently we have more than one lakh brands available in the market and inventory is always a big challenge for the community pharmacists. Selection of the medicines in the pharmacy primarily depends upon the flow of the prescriptions, patients, seasons, and visit of the medical representatives.

Determining the Quantity Required

Determination of the quantity is very important in the inventory process. Right quantity ensures the prescription honor, good sales and increased customer patronage. Quantity often depends upon the demand of the product, minimum purchase stock, discounts offered, availability of funds, and seasons etc.

Pharmacists should consider the stock types and requirements before placing an order in the following types.

(a) *Cycle stock:* Inventory for normal orders

(b) *Buffer or safety stock:* Additional stocks needed to meet the fluctuations

(c) *Anticipatory or speculative stock:* To meet the future demands or in case chances of price rise.

Procurement of Medicines

In routine practice, pharmacists place orders either by telephone, mail, fax, sales persons or through the medical representatives in the company order form. Generally the pharmacist or pharmacy assistant or owner of the pharmacy checks the stocks every day and makes list of the items to be procured from various suppliers based on the reorder level. Normally if the pharmacy is within the close vicinity of the supplier, the ordered items will be supplied on the same day. Otherwise the supplies will be made once a week or twice a week by the supplier. However the other factors that influence the procurement of the medicines are the urgency of the product, discounts or product deals, distance between the supplier and the pharmacy.

Selection of the Supplier

Supplier selection is very important in the procurement of the medicines. Attaining the right product at the right time and in the right place depends upon the right supplier. In order to rate the supplier, following criteria may be applied.

- Price
- Delivery methods and consistency
- Quality products and services
- Reliability
- Technical capability
- Financing and credit options

- Communication system
- Reputation in industry
- Attitude
- Customer service
- Geographical location
- Product return policy
- Assistance with product layout

The pharmacist can choose a supplier based on the feedback from other pharmacy owners and also with his past experiences.

Contract Terms

The contract terms have to be decided before a transaction begins. This includes the mode of payment, the schedule for payment, the time required for delivery of ordered medicines, etc.

Monitoring the Order Status

After the placement of the order, the pharmacist should monitor the order delivery status to avoid the stock out situations.

Check the Received Medicines

Once the ordered medicines have arrived at the pharmacy, they should be first quarantined and kept segregated from the usual shelf stocks, until they are verified with the given order and found correct. The stock has to be checked and tallied against the invoice for

- Name of the medicine.
- Strength of the medicine.
- Dosage form.
- Quantity of medicines received.
- Batch number.
- Expiry date.
- Cost price and taxes.
- Product discounts etc.

The medicines requiring cold chain have to be checked for storage during transit and quickly placed in the refrigerator. Newly ordered medicines should be checked for the expiry date. Typically newly arrived stock may have longer expiry date. So they should be placed behind the old stock. Stock rotation is a key principle in the inventory management to avoid expiries and unnecessary losses.

Payments to the Vendors

Payment should be made as specified in the contract. Prompt and reliable payment creates a good image for the pharmacy and pharmacist in the market and vendors will give preference to such clients for supplying the stocks.

Storage of Medicines

Procured medicines have to be stored appropriately at suitable temperature and humidity for long shelf life.

Product List

Product list is the list of medicines approved to be procured and stocked for sale in the pharmacy. This list contains all the information pertaining to the generic equivalents and brands, pack size, manufacturer, local distributor, with minimum and maximum reorder levels and reorder quantities. Approved product list helps the junior staff to place the orders in absence of senior staff.

Order List

An order list is the list of medicines to be ordered to the respective supplier with the required quantities based on the prescription demand. Appropriate quantities ordered in suitable time will help in minimizing the procurement costs. Order list depends upon the following factors such as

(a) Average daily/monthly consumption list
(b) Prevailing epidemics
(c) Seasonal diseases
(d) Regular patients with chronic ailments
(e) Company promotion schemes
(f) Regular sales call to physician by medical representative

Advantages of Inventory Control

The advantages of effective inventory control are

(a) Smooth flow of the goods to the pharmacy
(b) Prevents stock out situations
(c) Provides an opportunity for good customer service
(d) Increased customer patronage
(e) Helps in proper finance management in the pharmacy
(f) Good profits

INVENTORY CONTROL METHODS

Various methods of inventory control are practiced to procure the medicines to the pharmacy to meet the day-to-day demands within the assigned budget without the stock out or over stock situations. Following are the methods of inventory control.

1. ABC analysis (Always Better Control method)
2. VED analysis (Vital, Essential and Desirable)
3. EOQ method (Economic Order Quantity)
4. Perpetual Inventory Method
5. Physical Inventory
6. Lead time
7. Open to buy budget system
8. Bin card system
9. Minimum stock level
10. Maximum stock level

Always Better Control (ABC) Analysis

ABC method of inventory control is also called as always better control method. This method is based on the cost of the medicines. Medicines can be classified based on the cost as high cost medicines, moderate cost medicines and low cost medicines. As per the ABC analysis, 'A' category items are costly items, B category items are moderate cost items and C category items are economical items. As per the investment, 75% of the total allocated budget will be spent on category A items, 20% of the budgeted amount should be spent on 'B' category items, and 5% of the budget should be spent on purchasing category 'C' items. For efficient management of category 'A' items, strict control should be exercised to avoid pilferage and other losses.

Vital, Essential and Desirable (VED) Analysis

VED analysis is more often used in the automobile industry. This method is based on how important a particular part is irrespective of its cost. In health care industry, irrespective of the cost how effectively the medicine saves the life is the basis for VED analysis. For example in case of pesticide poisoning, to reverse the cholinergic symptoms, Atropine injection (Anti cholinergic agent) is commonly administered. Cost of the Atropine injection ranges between Rs.3-5/-. Since this medicine is vital in saving the life, thus it is called as Vital. The essential medicines are necessary to reduce the symptoms of a clinical condition such as Acid Pepsin Disease. In this clinical condition, proton pump inhibitors such as Omeprazole or Pantoprazole decreases the excess acid secretion and reduce the clinical condition. Thus such medicines are called as essential. Many water soluble vitamins (B-Complex) are available in food resources. Eating nutritious diet will supplement the adequate quantity of such vitamins. Thus B complex vitamins can be classified as desirable category.

Economic Order Quantity (EOQ) Method

Economic Order Quantity is one of the best known inventory models that are commonly utilized in purchasing the medicines for pharmacy. Economic Order Quantity (EOQ) is defined as the optimum quantity to be ordered at once. For ordering every product, it carries fixed ordering and procurement costs regardless of the number of units ordered. When the demand for a particular product is uniform round the year, if more numbers of orders are placed will attract more ordering costs and procurement costs. In order to minimize such costs without affecting the demand and supply, possible minimum numbers of orders are required to be placed. The minimum number of units placed in each order is called as Economic Order Quantity. This can be calculated by using the following formula.

$$\mathbf{EOQ} = \frac{\sqrt{2} \times PC \times Q}{CC}$$

PC = Procuring cost

CC = Carrying Cost

Q = Quantity of the product ordered in number of units

Procuring Cost includes communication expenditure, media cost, cost made on purchasing, receiving and checking goods, marking and stocking of goods.

Carrying Cost includes expenditures incurred due to the storage, insurance, interest on loan, deterioration of products or damage during the storage etc.

Perpetual Inventory Control Method

Perpetual inventory control method is a most effective and accurate method of inventory control. It is defined as the system of inventory control in which the number of units of any inventory item on any day can be obtained from the stock records. In this method all purchases and sales or consumption are recorded in inventory cards as they occur to provide a running balance of quantity and cost of items. As the items are counted daily or weekly or monthly basis every item will be physically counted at least once. If there is any mismatch due to human error, leakage, pilferage, loss between the physical quantity and the quantity shown in inventory cards, the records can be adjusted accordingly. With the use of computers, the work has become more simplified and the actual stock levels can be known at any point of time. It is very important to check and update the orders into computers to prevent the duplication.

Physical Inventory

Physical inventory is the physical verification of the stocks on weekly or monthly basis to identify the non moving items, stocks closing towards expiry, dead stock. Based on the information, the non moving stocks can be replaced with the supplier for fast moving items.

This will help both the supplier and the retailer in preventing the expiries. In physical inventory, the pharmacist can identify and prevent the pilferages and spoilages.

The stock position can be recorded in separate inventory sheets. Following is the model Inventory sheet for reference.

Model Inventory Sheet
Health Care Pharmacy
Naidu Nagar, Mysore

S.No.	Name of the Medicine	Package description	Qty	Price	Batch No.	Exp. Date	Total Value
1	MOX-500 Amoxicillin	15 Caps/Strip	22 units	Rs.140/unit	A-2309	May 15	3080 = 00
	MOX-250	15 Caps/Strip	18 units	Rs. 85/unit	K-3481	June 15	1530 = 00

Entered By:
Verified By:
Checked By:
Date:

Lead Time

Lead time is defined as the time gap between placement of an order to the supplier and actual receipt of the stocks. Lead time is the combination of ordering time, delivery time, and actual receipt of stocks.

Lead Time = Ordering time + Delivery time + Receiving Time

Ordering Time

Ordering time is the time taken to place an order. This depends upon the factors like selection of supplier, assessing the product demand, supply terms and discounts.

Delivery Time

Delivery time is time taken by the supplier in receiving the order from the chemist, separation of items, billing, packing, and choosing the right transport method to supply the stocks to the chemist. Delivery time may be influenced by the non availability of the ordered stocks with the distributor and lack of adequate clerical staff.

Receiving Time

Receiving time is the time taken to receive the supplied stocks from the wholesaler. Receiving time depends upon the transport system. If the pharmacy is located in a rural area and has poor transport system, the receiving time will increase. Thus such pharmacies require ordering excess stocks to meet the customer demand. Thus order quantity depends based on the above variables. Pharmacist should use his/her experience and expertise and acumen in ordering the suitable quantity to meet the market demand.

Open to Buy Budget System

Open to buy budget system is another method of inventory control commonly practiced in hospitals. In the preparation of the hospital budget, based on the previous year's sales record a stipulated amount is allocated as pharmacy budget for pharmacy requirements. Based on the sales requirement, the pharmacy manager will order the stock and the amount will be debited to the account. In this method the pharmacy manager will know the unwanted stock purchases and minimize the over stock and stock out situation.

Bin Card System

Bin Card system is a most simple and reliable method of inventory control. In this method, a separate card sheet is prepared for every product. The card contains the details such as manufacturer's name, date of supply, price, stock quantity, daily sales etc. In bin card system, the details should be updated on daily basis to get the accurate stock position and also helps the pharmacist to follow First In First Out (FIFO) system to liquidate the old stock.

KEY POINTS

- Efficient inventory control practices are essential to increase the customer patronage and maximize the profits of the pharmacy.
- Right product, right price, right vendor, and right time play as key elements for successful inventory.
- Always Better Control (ABC) method and Economic Ordering Quantity (EOQ) are the suitable inventory methods in procuring the medicines for community pharmacies.

SUGGESTED READINGS

1. Hyma P Gogineni, The fundamentals of pharmacy purchasing and inventory management. http://www.iarx.org/IowaPharmacy/Events.
2. Carroll, Norman V. Financial Management for Pharmacists: A decision making Approach. Philadelphia: Wolters Kluwer/Lippincot Williums and Wilkins. 2007.
3. American Society of Health System Pharmacists. ASHP guidelines on managing drug product shortages in hospitals and health systems. *Am J Health System Pharm.* 2009.66: 1399-406.

CHAPTER 10

OTC MEDICATION

LEARNING OBJECTIVES

- Define OTC medication.
- Know the process of converting a prescription drug to an OTC medicine.
- Appreciate the list of medicines available as OTC in various countries.
- Know the counseling points for various OTC medicines.

INTRODUCTION

Feeling unwell and suffering from minor ailments is a very common experience by individuals in all over the world. Majority people treat their ailments through self care using home remedies or over the counter (OTC) medicines. According to a worldwide review of consumer survey, about 50% of individuals either wait for the problem to run its course or use a home remedy. Another 25% the people visit a doctor or use a prescription medicine previously obtained for the same condition and the remaining 25% of the people visit the pharmacies to take OTC medicines.

Self-medication is the selection and use of medicines by individuals to treat self recognized minor ailment or symptoms. Self medication is an age old practice all over the world. The World Health Organization (WHO) promotes practice of self-medication for effective and quick relief of symptoms where medical services are inaccessible in rural and remote areas. Self medication with OTC medicines is sometimes referred as 'responsible' use of medicines. Self medication is widely practiced in both developed and developing countries. Over The Counter (OTC) medicines may be approved as being safe for self-medication by the national drug regulatory authority for prevention or treatment of minor ailments such as common cold, diarrhea, period pains, or symptoms which do not require immediate medical consultation.

Over The Counter (OTC) medicines are defined as "the medicine, or a pharmaceutical product, or drug, which is considered to be safe and effective in controlling the symptoms of minor ailments and can be sold to the customers by pharmacist without a valid prescription".

In some countries, medicines are categorized in to (a) Prescription Medicines, which are to be dispensed on a valid prescription, (b) Pharmacist only Medicines, which may be dispensed by the pharmacists depending upon the clinical judgment made by the pharmacists to treat minor ailments and (c) OTC medicines are the medicines available in pharmacies, groceries, and other shopping places to dispense for simple minor ailment such as headache and fever.

Advantages of having OTC Medicines List

Following are the advantages of having OTC medicines list.

- OTC medicines are considered to be safe and effective as they are approved by regulatory authority.
- Does not require a medical consultation thus saves the consultation charges to the patients.
- As the OTC medicines are deregulated from prescription status, the cost of the medicine may be economical.
- Waiting time for consultation is saved.
- Pharmacist can dispense OTC medicine without a prescription.

Examples of minor ailments and OTC medicines used to treat the minor ailments

Some examples of medical conditions that can be treated with over the counter drugs

- Nasal Allergies – Claritin, Benadryl
- Athlete Foot - Clotrimazole, Lamisil
- Cough and Cold - Guaifenesin DM, Mucinex DM
- Fever - Acetaminophen, Ibuprofen
- Migraine - Ibuprofen, Excedrin
- Pain and Inflammation - Ibuprofen, Naproxen
- Stomach Reflux - Ranitidine, Omeprazole

PROCEDURE TO SWITCH A PRESCRIPTION MEDICINE TO OTC MEDICINE

The reclassification of medicinal products from sale on prescription only to non prescription (over the counter or OTC) sale is of great current interest in many countries. Drug regulatory and health authorities have to consider the types of medicinal product for which reclassification is appropriate, safe and rational in the interest of public health. The transition of prescription drugs (Rx) to over-the-counter (OTC) status is a very complex and multifaceted process involving industry, regulatory authorities and health care professionals. The initiative for the review of prescription product as OTC medication generally will be taken by the pharmaceutical industry in the form of documented proposal to national drug regulatory authority. The drug regulatory authority will take suitable steps to reclassify the medicinal products as OTC medication. In some situations, products have been changed back from self-medication to prescription drug status due to new safety concerns.

Regulatory assessment of a change from prescription to non prescription status should be based on medical and scientific data on safety and efficacy of the compound and rationality in terms of public health. If a prescription product meets the few basic criteria such as, rationality of indications of a prescription substance support as OTC, provision of reliable and consistent relief of symptoms, favorable benefit/risk ratio of the product, wide safety margin even if used incorrectly, potentially less risks in comparison with prescription drugs that are commonly used in the same patient group, unaltered pharmacokinetics, low or well-characterized incidence of adverse effects or side effects, high safety profile in pregnancy and lactation, low level of drug dependence and abuse potential of the drug, existence of the other dosage forms of the same active ingredient that have already been approved for OTC sale, one or more specific routes of administration, dosage forms and formulations, the following additional criteria may favor consideration of change of status to non prescription sale:

1. The use of the product has been sufficiently extensive or in high volume.
2. The product has been marketed on prescription for at least five years. The time considered appropriate for a product to have been on prescription varies widely.

   E.g.: No time limit is specified in European union, three years in New Zealand, six years in Japan and up to ten years in Philippines.
3. Its adverse events give no cause for concern, and their frequency has not increased unduly during the marketing period.

Approved OTC Medicines List

Various countries have used World Health Organization (W.H.O) Anatomical, Therapeutic and Chemical (ATC) classification system and identified the medicines suitable as OTC medicines. A separate list of the medicines approved as OTC is published in majority of countries.

ROLE OF COMMUNITY PHARMACIST IN DISPENSING OTC MEDICINES

Pharmacists have a greater responsibility in educating the patients regarding safe use of medicines and monitor their health in terms of therapeutic outcomes and improved quality of life. Often patients visit pharmacies with enquiries about the management of minor ailments such as head ache, sore throat, stuffy nose and cough, diarrhea, period pains and body aches. Whenever the pharmacist dispenses the medicine, counseling about the non prescription medicines is very essential due to their potential interaction with disease process or with other prescription medicines. The pharmacist should ask the patient about the clinical condition for which the OTC medicine is required and also about the other prescription medicines the patient is taking. For example if a patient is suffering from stuffy nose and want a remedy for the clinical condition and the patient is hypertensive and taking antihypertensive medicines it is essential to avoid giving anticold preparation containing phenyl propalamine as this drug may elevate the blood pressure. Similarly if patient is using ciprofloxacin antibiotic and ask for an antacid for his acidity, if the pharmacist knows about the use of ciprofloxacin, the pharmacist may advice the patient to keep a gap of two hour between two drugs to prevent the absorption interaction and improve the therapeutic outcomes of both the drugs.

Specific Counseling Points for various Classes of OTC Medicines

Non Steroidal Anti-inflammatory Drugs (NSAIDs)

Non steroidal anti-inflammatory drugs (NSAIDs) such as Paracetamol, Ibuprofen, Diclofenac sodium are commonly used as OTC to treat fever, headache, muscle spasms, body and joint pains. These medicines are more potential to cause gastric irritation and continuous usage may precipitate as acid pepsin disease. These drugs also have the property to cause renal damage. To prevent the adverse effects associated with the use of NSAIDs, the patient should be given the following points.

- Take the medicine along with food and drink plenty of water.
- If intended relief is not felt with few doses, it is advisable to consult the doctor for further evaluation.
- If you are an asthmatic it is better to take such medicines under the supervision of a medical doctor.
- If you are using Aspirin, please consult the doctor for further use of Ibuprofen or Diclofenac.
- Tell your doctor if you have any allergies to your medicine.
- Store your medicines in a suitable box and keep it away from the children.
- If certain side effects such as confusion, swelling of face, feet or lower leg or sudden decrease in urine output is observed, contact the doctor immediately.
- You also inform your doctor about using these medicines as OTC. As these drugs have life threatening interactions with other drugs, your doctor may avoid them while prescribing.

Counseling Points associated with Use of Antibiotics

Antibiotics are the drugs that are used to treat infections caused by bacteria. These drugs are supposed to be taken for full course of time that is 5-7 days to cure the infection completely. Thus these drugs are to be taken under the medical supervision. Your doctor may choose the correct antibiotic based on your clinical condition.

- Take them as advised in right timings.
- Store them in suitable containers at appropriate temperature.
- Keep the medicines out of the reach to the children.
- If any adverse effects are seen, please contact your doctor immediately.
- If you have missed a dose, please take as soon as possible but do not double the dose which may be toxic.

- To know the potential drug interactions and adverse effects, please consult your pharmacist for suitable advice.

Counseling Points for using the Anti Cold and Cough Suppressants

Cold and cough suppressants are the agents used to give relief of symptoms associated with cold and flu such as sneezing, stuffy nose, itchy cough etc.

Following are the counseling points associated with anti cold and cough suppressing agents.

- These medicines may cause drowsiness, patients should be advised not to drive any vehicle or operate any heavy machinery.
- These medicines may cause dryness of mouth, nose and throat. For temporary relief use sugar less candy or gum or melt bits of ice cubes in the mouth.
- The decongestant medicines may cause restlessness or trouble in sleeping. Such people should be advised to take last dose of this medicine few hours before the bed time.
- As these medicines may pass through breast milk, nursing mothers should be advised to stop feeding the baby and give dairy milk.
- If you are taking any of these medicines such as CNS depressants, or MAO inhibitors please discuss with your doctor.

KEY POINTS

- OTC medicines play an important role in self care for minor ailments.
- Upon the request from pharmaceutical industry, regulatory authority converts the prescription status of a medicine to OTC medicine reviewing its safety and efficacy.
- Worldwide many countries have their own official OTC medicines list.
- Role of pharmacist is very much appreciated in the selection of the OTC medicines considering the patient's clinical conditions and prescription medicines the patient is already using.

SUGGESTED READINGS

1. Advice for the patient. Drug information in lay language. USPDI, 25th edition.
2. http://www.pharmaceutical-drug-manufacturers.com/pharmaceutical-drugs/non-prescription-drugs.html accessed on 25/10/2013
3. http://www.essentialdrugs.org/indiadrug/archive/200912/msg00008.php
4. http://www.catalystrx.com/www/shared/docs/mcs/MCS_2011_OTC_Medication_%20 Guide.PDF.

CHAPTER **11**

COMMUNICABLE DISEASES

LEARNING OBJECTIVES

- Know the causative organism
- Understand the clinical presentations of various communicable diseases
- Learn the strategies to prevent the communicable diseases

INTRODUCTION

Infection is defined as "the invasion of host organism by a pathogen such as virus, bacteria, fungi, nematodes, and other parasites by multiplication and releasing toxins causing the clinically evident illness". If such infections when spread from one person to other person are called as communicable diseases.

A communicable disease is defined as "an illness transmitted through contact with microorganisms". People, animals, food, surfaces, and air can all act as carriers of the microorganisms that pass infectious illnesses from one host to the next. The exchange of fluids or contact with a contaminated substance or individual may be sufficient enough to allow a communicable disease to spread.

Health promotion is defined as a combination of interventions such as health education and related organizational, economical and political interventions that promote the public health. Pharmacists are very important members of health care team and are in ideal position to play key role in ameliorating the public health.

In this chapter information is provided to understand causative pathogens, their clinical manifestations and prevention strategies of various communicable diseases causing concern to public health.

AMOEBIASIS

Introduction

Amoebiasis is an intestinal infection caused by a protozoa called as *Entamoeba histolytica*. It often spreads due to poor sanitation, contaminated food and drinking water. It is estimated that amoebiasis is the third most common cause of death caused by parasitic infections after schistosomiasis and malaria. In developing countries the infection rate is 30-40% and high in urban slums. In India, the prevalence rate of the infection is roughly around 15%.

Etiopathogenesis

The organism usually exists in two forms-the dividing form i.e., trophozoite and the dormant form i.e., the cyst. Human infection usually begins with the ingestion of the cyst that is present in contaminated food and water. Cysts survive in the acidic pH of the stomach and passes into the intestine. In the ileo-cecal region, cysts undergo excystment and each cyst gives rise to eight trophozoites. The trophozoites are 20 to 60 micrometer in diameter and contain vacuoles and a nucleus with a characteristic central nucleolus. The trophozoites migrate to colon for multiplication. In majority infected individuals, trophozoites live in the intestine as commensals. However trophozoites occasionally attack and invade the intestinal mucosa causing dysentery. The flask shaped ulcers are developed in ceacum and ascending of the colon. The trophozoites progress through the blood vessels to extra-intestinal locations like liver, brain and lungs and may form life-threatening abscesses. In the intestine, many of the trophozoites encyst and produce quadri nucleated cysts. Both trophozoites and cysts are excreted along with the feces. Cysts can survive for prolonged periods outside the host while the trophozoites survive few hours only. Trophozoites play no role in transmission of the disease but are responsible for producing tissue pathology. The reservoir of amebic infection is the asymptomatic human host or 'carrier' who continuously passes cysts. A carrier may excrete 15 million cysts per day.

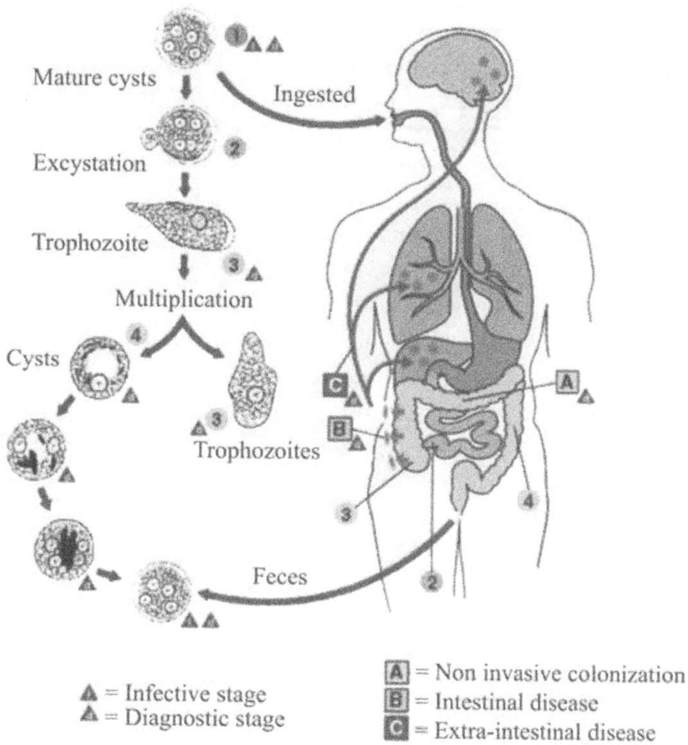

Clinical Features

In majority of the cases, infected individuals are asymptomatic. The symptoms of the infection include

- Fever.
- Abdominal discomfort and pain.
- Diarrhea containing blood or mucus.
- Offensive odor.
- Diarrhea alternating with periods of constipation or remission.
- Irregular bowel pattern.
- Ulceration of the skin (usually in the perianal region).
- Penile lesions in men after insertive anal intercourse.

The complications of amoebiasis include liver abscess or amoebic hepatitis. The symptoms of amoebic liver are pain in right upper quadrant abdomen, mild to moderate grade fever, poor general health and hepatomegaly.

Diagnosis

The diagnosis is mainly done by placing a small sample of stools under the microscope for the presence of the trophozoites and cysts. Microscopic stool examination from a single stool sample is only up to 50% sensitive but examination of 3 stool samples (taken over a period of up to 10 days) improves the sensitivity to 85-95%. In case of complications where there is suspicion of complications to liver and small intestine, ultrasound, computerized tomography (CT) scan and magnetic resonance imaging (MRI) scans of the abdomen are useful. In some cases, proctoscopy, sigmoidoscopy or colonoscopy and mucosal scrapings for biopsy are also done for confirmation of the pathogen.

Treatment

During ameobic dysentry, electrolyte replacement and nutritional support are essential adjunctive treatment modalities. The patient should be properly hydrated and should be given with oral re-hydration salts if there is severe dehydration. Large hepatic abscess or amoebic pericarditis may require needle aspiration, percutaneous catheter drainage, or rarely, surgery before drug therapy. Most regimens require a combination of drugs administered concurrently or sequentially.

The antiameobic agents are classified in to two groups. They are

- ***Luminal amoebicides***

  E.g., Iodoquinol, Diloxanide Furoate and Paromomycin.

- ***Tissue acting amoebicides***

  E.g., Metronidazole, Tinidazole, Tetracycline, Dihydroemetine, and Chloroquine.

The luminal amoebicides are very important because it is necessary to eradicate the causative agent from the lumen to prevent intestinal amoebiasis or the development of amoebic liver abscess.

Based on the Ministry of Health and Family Welfare of India guidelines, number of different regimens has been suggested depending on the category of amebiasis such as intestinal amoebiasis, amoebic liver abscess and asymptomatic cyst passers.

For Intestinal and Amoebic Liver Abscess

Metronidazole 800 mg three times a day orally for one week is recommended (35-40 mg/kg body weight given in 3 divided doses). In case if the patient is unconscious or in emergency condition administer 500 mg metronidazole through intravenous route. The other option is to administer tinidazole 2 grams once daily for 3 days (in mild to moderate infection) or 5 days (for severe infection). Diloxanide furoate 500 mg is given three times a day for 10 days (20 mg/kg body weight given in 3 divided doses).

For Intestinal Amoebiasis that has not Responded to Metronidazole and Diloxanide Therapy

In situation, where the patient has not responded to the metronidazole and diloxanide therapy, tetracycline 500 mg four times a day may be added for 5 days followed by 250 mg four times a day for 5 days (tetracycline 25-30 mg/kg body weight is given in 4 divided doses). The tetracycline therapy should be avoided during pregnancy and lactation.

For Amoebic Liver Abscess not Responding to Metronidazole

Chloroquine 250 mg tablet (containing 150 mg base), 2 tablets two times a day for 2 days followed by one tablet two times a day for 19 days (Chloroquine, 10 mg base/kg body weight for 2 days followed by 5 mg base/kg body weight for the next 19 days) is recommended.

Or, the other treatment option is dihydroemetine at a dose of 1 to 1.5 mg/kg body weight per day for 5 days. The maximum dose of dihydroemetine per day is 90 mg.

For Asymptomatic Cyst Passers

Iodoquinol is the drug of choice for the eradication of cysts. For adults the dose of iodoquinol is 650 mg three times a day for three weeks. For children, the dose is calculated at 10 mg/kg body weight given three times a day for 20 days. The maximum dose of iodoquinol should not exceed 2 grams per day.

Patient Education

About the Disease

- Amoebiasis is a disease which is caused by *Entamoeba hystolytica* a pathogen gets in to the stomach when contaminated food or drinking water is consumed.
- It is a communicable disease but curable.

- The commonly associated symptoms are abdominal pain, uneasiness, and diarrhoea with blood and mucus in stool.
- More severe illness occurs in children (especially neonates), people who are malnourished, patients whose immunity levels are less [E.g., Acquired Immune Deficiency Syndrome (AIDS) patient, cancer patient], pregnancy and post-partum.
- If adequate treatment is not taken, patients may end up in complications related to liver, intestine.

About the Medications

- Patient should be advised to take the medications regularly as per the doctor's advice. Patient should be informed not to miss any of the doses or discontinue any medicines after getting a temporary relief.
- Whenever the patient forgets to take the dose, advise the patient to take the dose as soon as he/she remembers. If it is time for the next dose, ask the patient to skip the previous dose. He/she should be advised not to double the dose.
- Specific antiprotozoal agents such as metronidazole, tinidazole, iodoquinol, diloxanide are often used to treat amoebiasis.
- Whenever the patient is using metronidazole or tinidazole, inform the patient that these medications may sometimes cause taste disturbances.
- Whenever the patient is using chloroquine and experiences palpitations or ringing sound in the ears, ask the patient to meet the doctor immediately. The other commonly associated adverse effects are headache, nausea.

About Life Style Modifications

- Patients suffering with the disease excrete the microbes in their stools which is likely to contaminate their hands and the environment. Thus they should be advised to take rest from work or school until they are symptom free.
- Patients should be advised to wash hands thoroughly with soap and running water after using the toilet or changing a baby's diaper, and before handling food.
- Patients should be advised to use clean bathrooms and toilets, a special attention should be given to toilet seats and taps. Patients should be educated to avoid sharing of towels.
- Do not consume milk, cheese or dairy products if they are not pasteurized.
- In rural areas, people should be educated not to pass their stools near the water bodies like rivers or lakes.
- During travel to the endemic areas, the visitors should be advised to drink packaged water only.

SYPHILIS

Introduction

Syphilis is a sexually transmitted disease caused by spirochete called *Treponema pallidum*. The organism is very small with a length of 6 to 20 μm and a diameter range of 18-20 μm. World Health Organization (WHO) estimated that more than 90% of the cases are occurring in developing countries. Recently syphilis has re-emerged in several developed countries like Russia, The United States, Canada, and England due to unsafe sex practices.

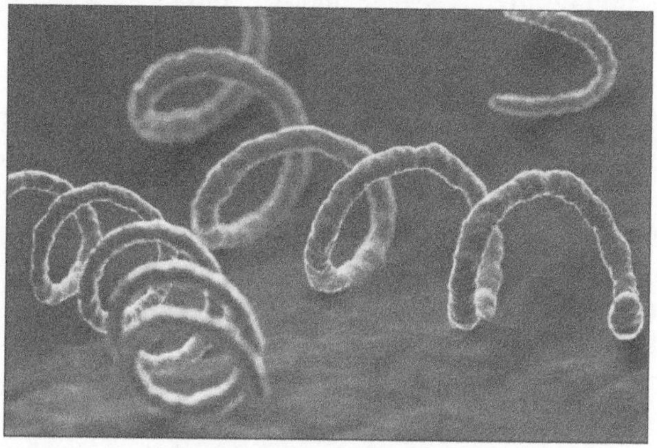

Treponema Pallidum

Mode of Transfer

(a) ***Sexual contact:*** The organism usually enters the body through broken skin or through the mucous membranes of the mouth, genitalia, or rectum during sexual contact. It can also be transmitted by kissing or intimate contact with an infected person.

(b) ***Non sexual contact:*** In rare occasions syphilis can be acquired by accidental inoculation or blood transfusion from an infected person. The disease can also be transmitted from an infected pregnant female to the foetus.

Pathogenesis

The incubation period varies from 10-90 days (usually 21 days) before the manifestation of the initial stages of syphilis. Syphilis is mainly divided into three stages depending upon the period after which the lesions appear, these are primary, secondary and tertiary.

(a) ***Primary syphilis:*** The typical lesion of primary syphilis is the appearance of an ulcer called 'chancre' usually associated with regional lymph node enlargement. The ulcer is usually single, painless, round and firm. The ulcer can be seen on ano-genital sites or at extra-genital sites like mouth and lips. The chancre lasts 3 to 6 weeks, and it heals without treatment. However, if adequate treatment is not administered, the infection progresses to the secondary stage.

(b) ***Secondary syphilis:*** This stage of syphilis usually develops after 2-3 months following primary syphilis. Secondary syphilis is the result of inadequately or untreated primary syphilis. The patients usually develop generalised lymph node enlargement along with cutaneous lesions and skin eruptions all over the body. The lesions are symmetric, pale red or pink, non pruritic, discrete, round that measure 5 to10 mm in diameter and are distributed on the trunk and proximal extremities. Some patients develop superficial mucosal erosions called ***mucous patches*** on mouth, palate, pharynx, glans penis and vagina. The mucous patches are usually pain less and silver grey in appearance. Antibody tests are always positive at this stage. This stage is highly infective stage and the spirochaetes can be easily demonstrated in the mucocutaneous lesions.

(c) ***Tertiary syphilis:*** This stage of syphilis usually develops after 2-3 years following secondary syphilis. The lesions of the tertiary syphilis are less infective and the organisms can not be detected very easily. The complications of tertiary syphilis are cardiovascular syphilis (chiefly affecting the aorta causing aortic aneurysm), neuro syphilis (chiefly affecting meninges, spinal chord or general paresis of the brain), and syphilitic gumma (solitary, localised, rubbery lesion with central necrosis) affecting organs like liver, testis, bone, brain.

Clinical Features

If the patient is in primary stage of the disease, soon after the incubation period, there will be appearance of an ulcer (chancre), usually with regional lymph node enlargement. The chancre may be present near the genital sites or on the extra genital sites like mouth, lips or tongue. The chancre will last for 3-6 weeks and heals without treatment.

If the patient is in the secondary stage of the disease, rashes will be seen in many parts of the body like hands, abdomen, feet, etc. These rashes are usually non-itching. In few patients, superficial mucosal erosions called *mucous patches* may develop on lips, oral mucosa, tongue, palate, pharynx, vagina and penis. A typical mucous patch is painless silver grey erosion surrounded by a red periphery.

Clinical Manifestations

Following are the clinical manifestations

- Rashes
- Fever
- Swollen lymph nodes
- Sore throat
- Headache
- Weight loss
- Muscle aches

In the late stages of syphilis, internal organs like brain, nerves, eyes, heart, blood vessels, liver, and bones also may get damaged in the patients. Signs and symptoms during this stage may be dementia, blindness, paralysis, numbness, widening and weakening of blood vessels like aorta (aneurysm of aorta).

Diagnosis

Treponema pallidum cannot be detected by culture test. Hence, the commonly used test is Dark-field microscopy which involves the examination of exudates from moist cutaneous lesions, such as the chancre of primary syphilis or the mucocutaneous lesions of secondary syphilis. Presence of characteristic motile organisms confirms the disease.

The second most commonly used test is Venereal Drug Research Laboratory (VDRL) test. It is a slide flocculation test. It mainly involves the usage of an antigen called 'cardiolipin' which is isolated from the beef heart. Patients suffering from syphilis produce antibodies those react with cardiolipin antigen which is similar to treponemal antigens and forms floccules. The patient's serum and cardiolipin are mixed in a cavity slide and rotated well for four minutes at suitable speeds (usually 180 rotations per minute). The slide is then viewed under the microscope for flocculation. Presence of floccules confirms syphilis. The VDRL test is also used for the diagnosis of neuro syphilis. Alternatively, other diagnostic tests used for syphilis detection are rapid plasma reagin test, Treponema pallidum Particle Agglutination (TP-PA) test and direct fluorescent antibody-*Treponema pallidum test.*

Management

Individuals with syphilis are at higher risk of acquiring other infectious diseases. All patients with syphilis should be assessed for other sexually transmitted diseases. Duration of treponemocidal level of antimicrobial should be at least 7-10 days to cover the dividing treponemes in early syphilis. Longer duration of treatment is needed as the duration of infection increases, possibly because of more slowly dividing treponemes in late syphilis.

Class	Drug	Dose	Route	Duration of use (days)
Penicillin	Benzathine Penicillin	2.4 million units	Intra muscular (1.2 million units each buttock) Or (2.4 units as a single injection)	01
	Procaine penicillin	600,000 units	Intra muscular	10-14
Cephalosporins	Ceftriaxone	500 mg	Intra muscular	10
Tetracyclines	Doxycycline	200 mg daily (either 100 mg twice daily or a single dose of 200 mg)	Oral	14
Macrolides	Tetracycline	500 mg	Oral	14
	Erythromycin	500 mg	Oral	14
	Azithromycin	2 gm	Oral	01

Penicillins

Penicillins are the first line agents used for treatment of syphilis. Parenteral route of administration is preferred rather than oral route because of guaranteed bioavailability. Long acting penicillins like benzathine penicillin 2.4 million units provides a treponemocidal penicillinaemia for upto 3-4 weeks (21-23 days). Benzathine penicillin is widely used because of efficacy and ease of treatment. Apart from benzathine penicillin, procaine penicillin in the dose of six lakh units for 10-14 days is also widely used. Replacing half of the solvent by 1% lidocaine solution may reduce the pain associated with injection and also improves the compliance. Newer anti treponemals include intramuscular or intravenous ceftriaxone. However there is significant cross reaction between cephalosporins and penicillin and anaphylaxis for penicillin is an absolute contraindication to the use of ceftriaxone.

***Non-penicillin** antibiotics used in the management of syphilis are:*

Tetracyclines like doxycycline, which is having good penetration into the CSF.

Macrolides like azithromycin and erythromycin. Azithromycin shows good anti-treponemocidal activity and studies have shown the effectiveness in the treatment of early syphilis. Erythromycin is least effective and does not penetrate the blood-brain or placental barriers well.

In the management of tertiary syphilis and treatment complications like syphilitic gumma, and cardiovascular syphilis the drugs should be used for a longer period of time. Benzathine penicillin is used in the dose of 2.4 million units intramuscular once weekly for three weeks (i.e., on days 1, 8 and 15). Procaine penicillin is used in the dose of 600,000 units intramuscular daily for 17-21 days. If the patient refuses penicillin administration or in case of penicillin allergies, the alternative drugs like doxycycline (200 mg per day either in single dose or in two divided doses) or tetracycline (500 mg four times a day) or erythromycin (500 mg four times a day) is recommended for 28 days.

Patient Education

About the Disease

- Syphilis is a disease which is caused by a pathogen called treponema.
- It is a communicable and multi stage disease but curable.
- The commonly associated symptoms are formation of ulcers (also called chancre) near the genital regions or near the mouth, lips etc., and these ulcers heal spontaneously without treatment. During the later stages of the disease, patient might experience rashes in one or more areas of the body usually on palms, hands, feet, abdomen, tongue, vagina etc., and these rashes are non itching. Along with these rashes a patient might also experience fever, malaise, weight loss, loss of appetite.

During the tertiary stages, the disease may further cause damage to internal organs like brain, blood vessels, nerves, bones and liver. During this stage the patient may experience difficulty in coordinating muscle movements, paralysis, numbness, gradual blindness, and forgetfullness.

- The risk factors associated with the development of syphilis are unprotected sexual practices, men having sex with men, hetero sexuality etc.

About the Medications

- Patient should be advised to take the medications regularly as per the doctor's advice and not to miss any of the doses and discontinue the medications after temporary relief. Whenever the patient forgets to take the dose of medications, advise the patient to take the dose as soon as he/she remembers and in case it is due for next dose advice them not to double the dose.
- If the patient is on penicillin injection, educate them that it can cause a bit pain due to its chemical structure.
- If a patient is allergic to penicillin antibiotics, he/she should be advised to stop the medicated anal consult his doctor for further course of action.
- If the patient is using tetracycline tablets, advice the patient not to consume milk, milk products or antacids together because these can reduce the activity of tetracycline. Advise the patient to take the tetracycline tablets and give a gap of two hours before consuming milk, milk products or antacids.
- If the patient has experienced any adverse effects such as headache, diarrhea and nausea patient should be advised to consult the doctor for further evaluation.

About Life Style Modifications

- If a person is diagnosed with syphilis immediately the partner also should be advised to get evaluated for the presence of the infection.
- Patients should be informed that there are no home remedies or over-the-counter drugs that can cure syphilis.
- It is important for the individuals to limit their sex partner to one to prevent the unwanted sexually transmitted infections.
- Patients should be advised to follow safe sex practices. They should be educated for proper usage of condoms which can avoid the spread of disease.
- Patients should be advised to use condoms lubricated with spermicides (especially Nonoxynol-9 or N-9) which is more effective in protecting against the transmission of sexually transmitted diseases than other lubricated condoms.
- If a person experiences any unusual discharge, sore or rash, particularly in the genital area, immediately he/she should avoid sex and consult a doctor immediately

TYPHOID

Introduction

Typhoid is an infectious communicable disease caused by various species of salmonella, especially *Salmonella typhi* and *Salmonella paratyphi*. Salmonella is a genus of gram negative bacteria that are the major cause of food borne illness throughout the world. Today, there are more than 2500 known species of salmonella. Typhoid continues to be a global health problem with an estimated 13 to 17 million cases worldwide resulting in 600,000 deaths per year. Typhoid fever is also called as "Enteric fever".

Causative Organism

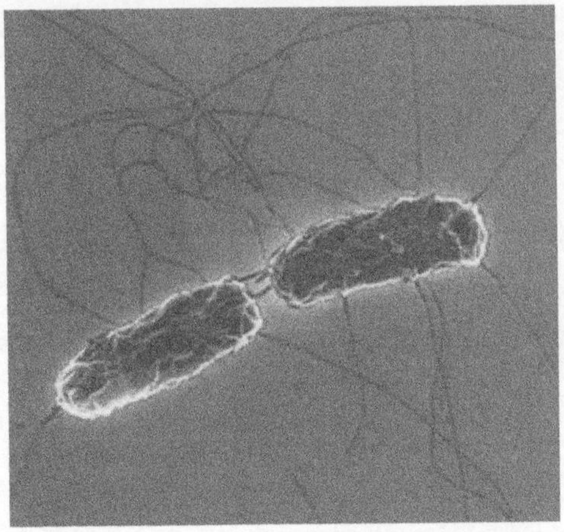

Salmonella typhi, Salmonella paratyphi

Mode of Transfer

The organisms usually enter the body through contaminated food or water, especially through faeces and contaminated beef and chicken that are insufficiently washed and cooked.

Pathogenesis

The incubation period varies from 5-14 days. The typhoid bacilli which are ingested through contaminated food or water are usually resistant to the gastric acid, following which they move to the intestine. They rapidly penetrate the mucosal epithelium and reach the lamina propria. The macrophages ingest the bacilli but do not generally kill them. Some bacilli remain within macrophages of the small intestinal lymphoid tissue. Other typhoid bacilli are drained into mesenteric lymph nodes where there is further multiplication and invasion of the lymphoid follicles and Peyer's patches (several lymph nodes near the junction of the ileum and colon) of the small intestine. Following this, the bacilli invade into the blood stream. The bacilli disseminate through out the body and colonize in reticuloendothelial tissues like liver, spleen, lymph nodes and bone marrow.

Clinical Manifestations

The commonly observed features of non complicated enteric fever are

- Prolonged high fever (103 -104 °F).
- Disturbances of bowel function (constipation in adults, diarrhoea in HIV patients and children).
- Headache.
- Malaise and anorexia.
- Cough is commonly seen in the early stage of the illness.
- During the period of fever, upto 25% of patients show exanthem (rose spots) on the chest, abdomen and back.

However, in severe and complicated cases, patients experience Melena (presence of blood in the faecal matter), intestinal perforations and peritonitis usually associated with abdominal discomfort, hypotension, marked abdominal tenderness and a rising white blood cell count.

Diagnosis

The diagnosis is mainly done by placing a small sample of blood, urine, stool or bone marrow in special medium that encourage the growth of bacteria. After 48-72 hours, the culture is checked under the microscope for the presence of typhoid bacteria. The commonly used media for blood samples are blood agar media and MacConkey agar media. The commonly used media for stool samples or rectal swabs are MacConkey agar media, Salmonella shigella agar media, Deoxycholate citrate agar media.

Apart from the above test, the most widely used serological test for diagnosis of typhoid fever is "Widal test". The test is named after a French physician and bacteriologist named Georges Fernand Isidore Widal. The basic principle of Widal test is that patients' suffering from typhoid fever would possess antibodies in their sera which can react and agglutinate with dilutions of killed, coloured salmonella antigens in a tube/slide. Blood samples are collected from the patients suspected with typhoid. The serum is separated and mixed with known amount of diluted salmonella antigens like *Salmonella typhi H* antigen, *Salmonella typhi* O antigen, *Salmonella paratyphi* AH antigen in separate tubes/slides.

The tubes/slides are maintained at 37 °C overnight and observed for the presence of any agglutination. Presence of agglutination confirms typhoid fever.

Treatment (Adopted from the WHO typhoid guidelines)

Supportive measures like oral rehydration, proper nutrition, and use of antipyretics are important in the management of typhoid fever. More than 90% of patients can be managed at home with oral antibiotics, reliable care and close medical follow-up for complications or failure to respond to therapy. However, patients with persistent vomiting, severe diarrhoea and abdominal distension may require hospitalization and initiation of parenteral antibiotic therapy.

Susceptibility	Optimal therapy			Alternative effective drugs		
	Antibiotic	Daily dose (mg/kg)	Days	Antibiotic	Daily dose (mg/kg)	Days
Fully sensitive	Fluoroquinolone (E.g., Ofloxacin or Ciprofloxacin)	15	5-7	Chloramphenicol Amoxicillin TMP-SMX*	50-75 75-100 8-40	14-21 14 14
Multidrug resistance	Fluoroquinolone Cefixime	15 15-20	5-7 7-14	Azithromycin Cefixime	8-10 15-20	7 7-14
Quinolone resistance	Azithromycin Ceftriaxone	8-10 75	7 10-14	Cefixime	20	7-14

*TMP-SMX: Trimethoprim-Sulfamethaxazole

The fluoroquinolones are optimal for the treatment of typhoid fever in adults. They are relatively inexpensive, well tolerated and more reliable than the previously used drugs like chloramphenicol, ampicillin, amoxicillin and trimethoprim-sulfamethoxazole. The fluoro quinolones attain an excellent tissue penetration and kill *S. typhi* in its intracellular stationary stage in monocytes/macrophages and achieve higher active drug levels in the gall bladder than other drugs. However, in some countries the use of fluoro quinolones is relatively contraindicated in children because of concerns that they may cause articular damage.

As an alternative therapy, ampicillin and amoxicillin are used at the dose of 500 mg per oral in three or four doses. No benefit has been reported due to the addition of clavulanic acid to amoxicillin. Trimethoprim-sulfamethoxazole, (TMP-SMZ) can be used orally in adults at a dose of 160 mg TMP plus 800 mg SMZ twice daily or in children at 4 mg TMP per kg and 20 mg SMZ per kg for 14 days.

For the treatment of resistant species, third-generation cephalosporins like oral cefixime (15-20 mg per kg per day, 100/200 mg twice daily) has been widely used. Recent data on azithromycin use in children indicate that it may be safely given as an alternative agent for the treatment of uncomplicated typhoid fever. Azithromycin in a dose of 500 mg (10 mg/kg) given once daily for seven days has proved effective in the treatment of typhoid fever in adults and children.

In case of severe and complicated cases intravenous antibiotics are required, ciprofloxacin or ofloxacin can be used (15 mg per kg per day for 7-14 days). Apart from the fluoroquinolones, cephalosporins may also be recommended in the following doses: ceftriaxone, 50-75 mg per kg per day (2-4 gm per day for adults) in one or two doses; cefotaxime, 40-80 mg per kg per day (2-4 gm per day for adults) in two or three doses; and cefoperazone, 50-100 mg per kg per day (2-4 gm per day for adults) in two doses.

The parenteral fluoroquinolones are probably the correct choice in severe infections. In severe typhoid the fluoroquinolones are given for a minimum of 10 days. Patients with typhoid fever showing changes in mental status, characterized by delirium, stupor should be immediately evaluated for meningitis by examining the cerebrospinal fluid. If the findings are normal and typhoid meningitis is suspected, the patients should be immediately treated with high doses of corticosteroid like dexamethasone (3 mg/kg as a slow intravenous infusion) in addition to the antimicrobials.

Patient Education

Community pharmacist may provide education to the patient about the disease and medications. Following are the patient counseling points.

About the Disease

- Typhoid is a disease which is caused by microbes (bacteria) called salmonella and is communicable but curable.
- The symptoms associated with typhoid are fever, abdominal pain, headache, uneasiness, vomiting, constipation or diarrhoea (adults tend to get constipation and children tend to get diarrhoea).
- The sources of infection for typhoid are improper hygiene, usage of improperly cooked food and meat, contaminated drinking water, etc.
- A small number of patients may experience typhoid fever complications such as intestinal ulcers, infections to heart, brain or even some times multiple organ failure.

About the Medications

- Patient should be advised to take the medications regularly as per the doctor's advice. Patient should be informed not to miss any of the doses or discontinue any medicines after experiencing the temporary relief.
- Whenever the patient forgets to take the dose of medications, advise the patient to take the dose as soon as he/she remembers. If it is time for the next dose, ask the patient not to double the dose as it can cause some harmful effects on the body.
- If the patient experiences any adverse effects with medicines, the patient should be advised to contact the pharmacist or doctor immediately.

About Life Style Modifications

- Patients suffering from the typhoid fever may excrete the microbes into their stools which are likely to contaminate the hands and the environment. They should be excluded from work or school until they become symptom free.
- Patients should be advised for general hygiene, they should be educated for washing and drying the hands after visiting the toilet and before handling the food.

MALARIA

Malaria is one of the major public health problems of the country. Malaria is caused by protozoan parasite *Plasmodium*. The parasites are inoculated into the human host by a female anopheles mosquito. The four *Plasmodium* species that infect humans are *P. falciparum, P. vivax, P. ovale* and *P. malariae.*

Etiopathogenesis

Human infection begins when a female anopheles mosquito inoculates plasmodial *sporozoites* from its salivary gland during a blood meal. These microscopic motile forms of the malarial parasites are carried rapidly *via* the bloodstream into the liver, where they invade hepatic parenchymal cells and begin asexual reproduction. By this amplification process (known as intrahepatic or pre erythrocytic *schizogony* or *merogony)* a single *sporozoite* eventually produce 10,000 to 30,000 daughter merozoites. The swollen liver cell eventually bursts, discharging motile *merozoites* into the bloodstream. The released merozoites invade the red blood cells (RBCs) and multiply 6 to 20 fold every 48 to 72 hr. When the parasites reach densities of 50/L of blood, the symptomatic stage of the infection begins. Intra hepatic forms do not divide immediately but remain dormant for a period ranging from 3 weeks to a year or longer in *P. vivax* and *P. ovale* infections. These dormant forms, or *hypnozoites*, are the cause for the relapses.

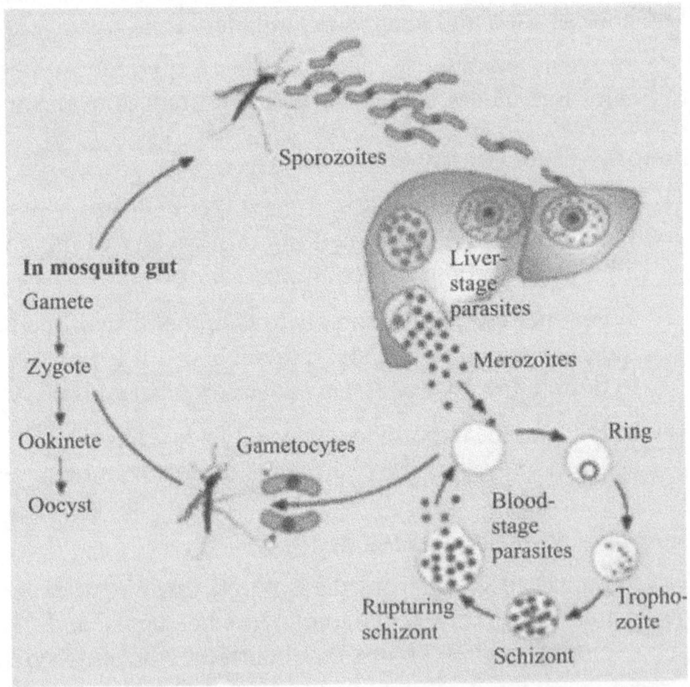

After entry into the bloodstream, *merozoites* rapidly invade erythrocytes and become *trophozoites*. Attachment is mediated *via* a specific erythrocyte surface receptor. During the early stage of intraerythrocytic development, the small 'ring forms' of the four parasitic species appear similar under light microscopy. As the trophozoites enlarge, species-specific characteristics become evident, pigment becomes visible, and the parasite assumes an irregular or amoeboid shape. By the end of the 48 hr intraerythrocytic life cycle (72 hr for *P. malariae*), the parasite has consumed nearly all the hemoglobin and grown to occupy most of the RBC. It is now called a *schizont*. Multiple nuclear divisions have taken place (*shizogony* or *merogony*), and the RBC ruptures to release 6 to 30 daughter *merozoites*, that are potentially capable of invading a new RBC and repeating the cycle. The disease in human beings is caused by the direct effects of RBC invasion and destruction by the asexual parasite and the host's reaction.

Life Cycle of malaria Paracyte

After a series of asexual cycles (*P. falciparum*) or immediately after release from the liver (*P. vivax*, *P. ovale*, *P. malariae*) some of the parasites develop into morphologically distinct, long-lived sexual forms (*gametocytes*) that can transmit malaria.

When female anopheles mosquito bites an individual, male and female *gametocytes* enter into the mosquito and form a *zygote* in the insect's midgut. This *zygote* matures into an ookinete, which penetrates and encysts in the mosquito's gut wall. The resulting *oocyst* expands by asexual division until it bursts to liberate myriad motile *sporozoites*, which then migrate in the hemolymph to the salivary gland of the mosquito to await inoculation into another human at the next feeding.

Clinical Features

Following are the clinical manifestations in malaria infection

- Intermittent fever
- Chills and rigors
- Headache
- Myalgia
- Arthralgia
- Anorexia
- Nausea and Vomiting

Malaria should be suspected in patients residing in endemic areas and presenting the above symptoms. It may also be suspected in patients who have recently visited to an endemic area. Although malaria is known to mimic the signs and symptoms of many common infectious diseases, the other causes should also be suspected and investigated in presence of the following manifestations.

- Running nose, cough and other signs of respiratory infection
- Diarrhoea/dysentery
- Burning micturition and/or lower abdominal pain
- Skin rash/infections
- Abscess
- Painful swelling of joints
- Ear discharge
- Lymphadenopathy

The following may be seen in severe Malaria

- Coma (cerebral malaria)
- Metabolic acidosis

- Severe anemia
- Hypoglycemia
- Acute renal failure or
- Acute pulmonary edema

Management of Malaria

To treat clinical malaria, chloroquine is the best option in the dose of 25 mg/kg per day for three consecutive doses. As per the WHO recommendations, for managing chloroquine sensitive malaria, 600 mg chloroquine base (4 tablets of chloroquine sulphate) followed by 300 mg chloroquine base after six hours followed by 300 mg chloroquine base every day for next three consecutive days.

WHO recommends that artemisinin-based combination therapies with different mechanisms of action for the treatment of chloroquine resistant uncomplicated *P. falciparum* malaria. The artemisinin derivative components must be given for at least three days for an optimum effect. Artemisinin and its derivatives should not be used as monotherapy.

Rationale for Antimalarial Combination Therapy

Antimalarial combination therapy (ACT) with simultaneous use of two or more schizontocidal agents with independent modes of action is only to target the parasite. The rationale for the combination is: i) the combination is often more effective; and ii) to kill the mutant parasite. This mutual protection is thought to prevent or to delay the emergence of resistance.

The Artemisinin based Combination therapy (ACT) Options now Recommended for Treatment of Uncomplicated Falciparum Malaria

- ***Artemether plus lumefantrine:*** This is currently available as a fixed-dose formulation with dispersible or standard tablets containing 20 mg of artemether and 120 mg of lumefantrine.

  Therapeutic dose: The recommended treatment is a 6-dose regimen over 3-days period.

- ***Artesunate plus amodiaquine:*** This is currently available as a fixed-dose formulation with tablets containing 25/67.5 mg, 50/135 mg or 100/270 mg of artesunate and amodiaquine.

  Therapeutic dose: A target dose of 4 mg/kg/day artesunate and 10 mg/kg/day amodiaquine once a day for 3 days, with a therapeutic dose range between 2-10 mg/kg/day artesunate and 7.5-15 mg/kg/dose amodiaquine.

- ***Artesunate plus mefloquine:*** This is currently available as blister packs with separate scored tablets containing 50 mg of artesunate and 250 mg base of mefloquine, respectively.

  Therapeutic dose: A target dose of 4 mg/kg/day artesunate given once a day for 3 days and 25 mg/kg of mefloquine either split over 2 days as 15 mg/kg and 10 mg/kg or over 3 days as 8.3 mg/kg/day once a day for 3 days. The therapeutic dose range is between 2-10 mg/kg/Dose/day of artesunate and 7-11 mg/kg/Dose/day of mefloquine.

- ***Artesunate plus sulfadoxine-pyrimethamine:*** This is currently available as separate scored tablets containing 50 mg of artesunate and tablets containing 500 mg of sulfadoxine and 25 mg of pyrimethamine.

  Therapeutic dose: A target dose of 4 mg/kg/day artesunate given once a day for 3 days and a single administration of 25/1.25 mg/kg sulfadoxine-pyrimethamine on day 1, with a therapeutic dose range between 2-10 mg/kg/day artesunate and 25-70/1.25-3.5 mg/kg sulfadoxine-pyrimethamine.
- ***Dihydroartemisinin plus piperaquine:*** This is currently available as a fixed-dose combination with tablets containing 40 mg of dihydroartemisinin and 320 mg of piperaquine.

  Therapeutic dose: A target dose of 4 mg/kg/day dihydroartemisinin and 18 mg/kg/day piperaquine once a day for 3 days, with a therapeutic dose range between 2-10 mg/kg/day dihydroartemisinin and 16-26 mg/kg/day piperaquine.

Second-line Antimalarial Treatments

On the basis of the evidence from current practice and the consensus opinion of the Guidelines Development Group, the following second-line treatments are recommended:

- Artesunate plus tetracycline or doxycycline or clindamycin (given for a total of 7 days)

  Therapeutic dose: Artesunate (2 mg/kg once a day) plus tetracycline (4 mg/kg four times a day) or doxycycline (3.5 mg/kg once a day) or clindamycin (10 mg/kg twice a day).

  Any of these combinations should be given for 7 days.
- Quinine plus tetracycline or doxycycline or clindamycin (given for a total of 7 days).

  The alternative ACT has the advantages of simplicity and improves the adherence. The 7-day regimens are not well tolerated and adherence is likely to be poor if treatment is not observed. It is essential that the patient and the caregiver understand the importance of completing the full 7-day course of treatment.

Treatment in Specific Populations and Situations

Pregnant Women

Pregnant women with symptomatic acute malaria are considered to be a high-risk group, and they must be promptly treated with a suitable and safe antimalarial drug. Malaria in pregnancy is associated with low birth weight, increased anemia and death.

First Trimester

- Quinine plus clindamycin to be given for 7 days (artesunate plus clindamycin for 7 days is indicated if this treatment fails).

- ACT is indicated only if this is the treatment available immediately, or if treatment with 7-day quinine plus clindamycin fails, or if there is uncertainty about patient compliance with a 7-day treatment.

Second and Third Trimesters

- ACT is known to be effective in the country/region or artesunate plus clindamycin to be given for 7 days or quinine plus clindamycin to be given for 7 days.

Lactating Women

Lactating women should also receive the recommended antimalarial treatment (including ACTs), except primaquine and tetracycline.

Infants and Young Children

ACTs should be used as first-line treatment for infants and young children with uncomplicated malaria, and careful attention should be paid to accurate dosing and ensuring the administered dose is retained. Young children cannot swallow antimalarial medicines reliably. So treatment with rectal artesunate may be recommended.

Travellers

For travelers going to non-endemic countries with uncomplicated malaria:

- Atovaquone plus proguanil [15/6 mg/kg (adult dose – 4 tablets) once a day for 3 days]
- Artemether plus lumefantrine
- Dihydroartemisinin plus piperaquine
- Quinine plus doxycycline or clindamycin

Patient Education

- Advice the travelers planning to visit the endemic areas about the infection, prophylaxis and also about preventive measures to avoid the mosquito bite.
- Help the patients to know about their medication, such as what for the medication was prescribed, dose, duration, potential side effects and strategies to prevent them.
- Motivate the patients to take the prescribed medicines regularly without fail and in case if a dose is missed, the patient should be advised not to miss the doses and not to double the dose if it is due for next dose.
- Advice patients to take suitable life style modification such as using mosquito nets, mosquito repellent creams to prevent re-infection.

ACQUIRED IMMUNE DEFICIENCY SYNDROME (AIDS)

Introduction

Acquired Immune Deficiency Syndrome (AIDS) was first described in 1981 as a new clinical entity and in 1983 the Human Immunodeficiency Virus (HIV) was considered as causative agent for AIDS. Human Immunodeficiency Virus is a retrovirus which is classified into HIV-1 and HIV-2 and depletes the helper T cells and causes opportunistic infections and malignancies. As per Joint United Nations Programme on AIDs (UNAIDs) estimates about 34 million people are living with HIV/AIDS. Majority of these patients come from Sub Saharan Africa, Asia, and South America. AIDS is characterized by progressive destruction of the body's immune system. The three primary modes of transmission responsible for HIV infection are sexual, parenteral, and perinatal. Receptive anal and vaginal intercourse is the most common route for HIV transmission as highest viral concentration is found in blood and seminal fluid. Individuals with genital ulcers or sexually transmitted diseases, such as syphilis, chancaroid, herpes, gonorrhea, chlamydia, and trichomoniasis, are at greater risk for contracting HIV. However, condom use reduces the transmission risk by approximately 20-fold.

Drug addicts sharing injection paraphernalia are at greater risk for HIV transmission. Healthcare workers also do possess small amount of risk of acquiring HIV due to accidental percutaneous needle stick injury. Vertical transmission or perinatal infection is the most common cause in pediatric HIV infection. The risk of mother-to-child transmission is approximately 40% in the absence of antiretroviral therapy and breast feeding. The amount of viral load in the woman at the time of delivery is key factor for vertical transmission. Infected blood and blood products also transmit HIV infection.

Morphologic Structure of HIV-1

Anatomy of the AIDS virus

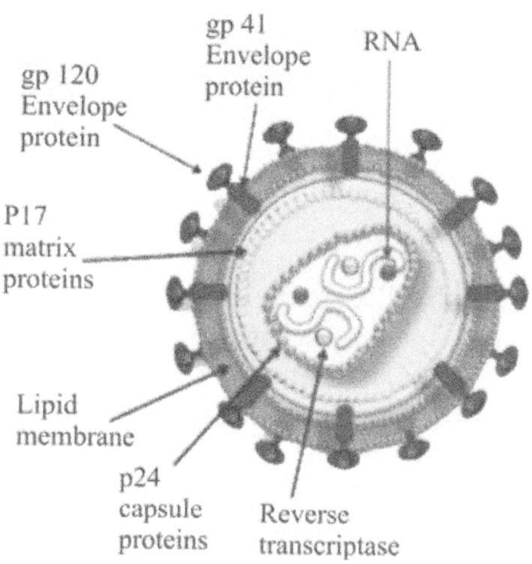

HIV-1 is a retrovirus belongs to family lentiviruses. The diameter of the HIV-1 viral particle is 100 nm and surrounded by a lipoprotein membrane. Each viral particle possesses 72 glyco protein complexes. Among them, the gp120 and gp41 are important proteins. The bond between gp120 and gp 41 are loose and gp120 is easily sheds and thus seen in the serum and lymphatic tissues of HIV infected patients. During the process of budding, the virus may incorporate HLA I and II class proteins and adhesion proteins (ICAM -1) for adhesion to target cell. The p17 is anchored to the inside of the viral lipoprotein membrane. The p24 core antigen contains two copies of HIV-1 RNA which is nucleoprotein p7 and the reverse transcriptase p66. The viral particle contains all the enzymatic equipment that is necessary for replication: a reverse transcriptase (RT), an integrase p32 and a protease p11.

Pathophysiology

The Human Immuno deficiency Virus attacks and binds to specific cells of the immune system, including monocytes, macrophages, and T-cell lymphocytes (also called as CD4+ T cells or helper T cells). The virus requires co-receptor proteins (CCR-5, CXCR-4) for fusion after binding to the CD4 cell. HIV fuses with the cell and releases its contents into the host cell's cytoplasm: this includes the virus' RNA and specific enzymes necessary for replication. Reverse transcriptase enzyme converts the single-stranded viral RNA into a double-stranded proviral DNA. The integrase enzyme incorporates proviral DNA into the host cell's genetic material. The virus uses the infected cell's machinery for translation and transcribing to produce immature viral particles which may bud and break from the infected cell. Upon maturation, the virion infects new host cells and subsequently produce more infections virus. The virus also may get destroyed by mechanisms such as direct cytolytic effect of the virus, the host's immune response (e.g., *via* cytotoxic T-cell lymphocytes) or due to the cell's natural life cycle coming to completion. Most infectious HIV virions (~99%) live inside the lymph nodes and other immune-cell rich tissues found throughout the body. The immune system reacts by producing antibodies against HIV however, given the rapid production of new HIV particles and the development of various new viral strains the antibody response is inadequate. After this burst of viremia, a transient depletion of CD4 cells occurs and patients complains of non specific symptoms such as fever, lymphadenopathy, rash, fatigue, and night sweats. This phase of infection is known as the acute retroviral syndrome. In most of the cases, the patients may not know about their infection status. Within 6 months, the host's immune response is able to control the infection to a point where the number of virus particles produced per day equals the number of particles destroyed per day. This steady-state is often referred to as the patient's viral "set point". Higher the patient's viral set point, greater will the risk for disease progression due to wide spread of the infections.

Clinical Presentations

Clinical presentations of primary HIV infection are

- Fever
- Pharyngitis
- Adenopathy

Probability of progression to acquired immune deficiency syndrome (AIDS) is related to RNA viral load. Center for Disease Control and Prevention classifies HIV infection into nine categories based on the CD4 cell count. Most children born with HIV are asymptomatic. On physical examination, they often present with unexplained physical signs such as lymphadenopathy, hepatomegaly, splenomegaly, failure to thrive, and weight loss or unexplained low birth weight, and fever of unknown origin.

Lab Investigations Elisa Test

Enzyme-Linked Immunosorbent Assay (ELISA) is commonly used screening method for HIV and detects antibodies against HIV-1. It is highly sensitive and specific. False positive result may be seen in multiparous women, individuals recently infected with hepatitis B, HIV, influenza and received rabies vaccine. False negative results may occur in newly infected patients before antibody production is adequate.

Western blot assay is the most commonly used confirmatory test. The viral load test quantifies viremia by measuring the amount of viral RNA. Other methods used for determining the amount of HIV RNA are reverse transcriptase-coupled polymerase chain reaction, branched DNA, and nucleic acid sequence-based assay. The normal adult CD4 lymphocyte count ranges between **500 and 1,600 cells/ml.**

WHO Disease Staging System

World Health Organization (WHO) classifies HIV infection into four stages.

Stage I: HIV infection is asymptomatic and not categorized as AIDS

Stage II: Includes minor mucocutaneous manifestations and recurrent upper respiratory tract infections

Stage III: Includes unexplained chronic diarrhea for longer than a month, severe bacterial infections and pulmonary tuberculosis

Stage IV: Includes the toxoplasmosis of the brain, candidiasis of the esophagus, trachea, bronchi, or lungs and kaposi's sarcoma which are the indicators of AIDS

Non Pharmacologic Management

HIV infected individuals do not show any clinical manifestations as long as the CD4+ count is within the normal range. Adequate life style modifications, nutritious diet help the infected individuals to maintain the adequate CD4+ count. Lifestyle modifications include limiting the sex partner to one, using the condom during the sex, preventing the use of blades and sharps used by other individuals, maintaining the personal hygiene, eating well cooked foods and well cleaned fruits, abstaining from alcohol, smoking tobacco and prevent self from situations that may worsen their condition.

Pharmacological Management

Preventing viral replication is the main strategy in HIV infection management. As per International AIDS society, Center for Disease and Prevention, World Health Organisation guidelines recommends three classes of antiretroviral agents to prevent the viral multiplication.

They are

1. **Nucleoside Reverse Transcriptase Inhibitors (NRTIs)**

   E.g., zidovudine, Didanosine, Stavudine, Zalcitabine, Lamivudine, Abacavir
2. **Non Nucleoside Reverse Transcriptase Inhibitors (NNRTIs)**

   E.g., Nevirapine, Delavirdine, Efavirenz
3. **Protease Inhibitors (PIs)**

   E.g., Saquinavir, Ritonavir, Indinavir, Nelfinavir, Amprenavir

Important goal of the antiretroviral therapy is the undetectable viral load. Strict adherence to the medication is important in therapeutic success. Suitable combination of antiretroviral agents is commonly used to prevent the resistance and drug failure.

Clinical category	CD4 T cell count and HIV viral load	Treatment recommendations	Treatment regimens
Symptomatic Unexplained fever Oral Thrush	Any value	Treat	2 NRTI + 1 PI 2 NRTI+ 2 PI 2 NRTI + 1 NNRTI 2 NRTI+1NNRTI + 1PI
Asymptomatic	CD 4 Count $< 500/mm^3$	Patient should be explained about the importance of anti retroviral agents	
Pregnancy	Any value	Treat mother and passively the fetus	Zidovudine should be added in maternal regimen
New Born	Any value and with high risk	All neonates, all infants born to HIV infected mothers will be HIV +	For neonates, 6 weeks of Zidovudine, 2 mg/kg 6th hrly beginning 1-8 hours of birth
Occupational and non occupational exposure prophylaxis		Treatment should be initiated within 72 hr of exposure	2 NRTI+ PI

Patient Education

Adherence to antiretroviral agents is the key element in the success of the HIV infection management. Many research studies have proved a direct relationship between the medication adherence and CD4+ count. Pharmacist has a significant role in improving the patients' understanding about the disease progression, importance of regular consumption of antiretroviral agents, healthy diet and lifestyle modifications. The community pharmacists should maintain the confidentiality of the serostatus of the patients to prevent any embracing situations to the patients.

GONORRHEA

Gonorrhea is sexually transmitted infection caused by *Neisseria gonorrhea*, a bacterium (gram negative, non-motile non spore forming) that grows and multiplies quickly in moist, warm areas of the body such as the cervix, urinary tract, mouth, or rectum.

Etiology

Men have a 20% chance of getting the infection by having sexual relations with a woman infected with gonorrhea. Women have a 50% chance of getting the infection by having sexual relations with a gonorrhea infected man.

Pathophysiology

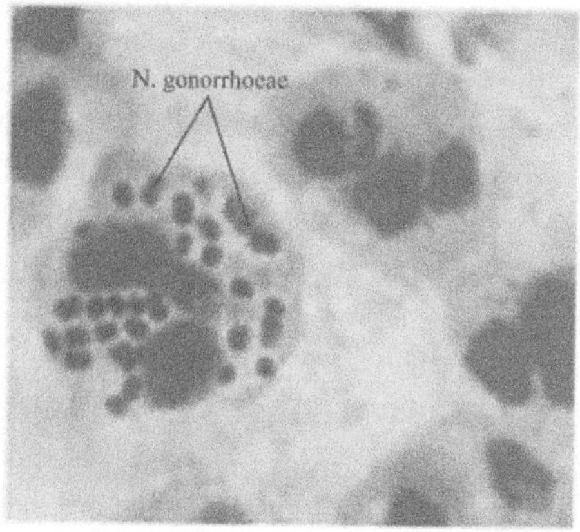

Gonorrhea primarily affects the epithelium and mucous membrane of lower genital tract; however it may also involve the eyes, oropharynx and anus. On contact with a mucosal surface (lined by columnar, cubouidal, or noncornified squamous epithelial cells), the gonococci attach to cell membranes by pili, one of the primary virulence factors, they are pinocytosed. After mucosal damage is established subsequently polymorphonuclear leukocytes invade the tissue, leading to secretion of purulent exudates.

Clinical Representation

Individuals infected with gonorrhea can be symptomatic or asymptomatic, it may be complicated or uncomplicated infections and it may be different in men and women.

In men	In women
General Incubation period 1-14 days	**General** Incubation period 1-14 days
Symptoms onset in 2-8 days	Symptoms onset in 10 days
Site of infection Urethra, rectum, oropharynx.	**Site of infection** Most common-endocervical anal, urethra, rectum, oropharynx, eye.
In men	**In women**
Symptoms • Abnormal discharge from the penis (clear or milky at first, and then yellow, creamy, and excessive, sometimes blood-tinged). • Painful or frequent urination or urethritis. • Anal itching, discomfort, bleeding, or discharge. • Sore throat (rare). • Pinkeye (conjunctivitis) (rare). .	**Symptoms** • Painful or frequent urination. • Anal itching, discomfort, bleeding, or discharge. • Abnormal vaginal discharge. • Abnormal vaginal bleeding during or after sex or between periods. • Genital itching. • Irregular menstrual bleeding. • Lower abdominal (belly) pain. • Fever and general tiredness. • Swollen and painful glands at the opening of the vagina (Bartholin glands). • Painful sexual intercourse
Complications Rare (epididymitis, prostatitis, inguinal lymphadenopathy, urethral structure)	Pelvic inflammatory disease and associated complications

Laboratory Studies

Culture is the most common diagnostic test for gonorrhea and then polymerase chain reaction (PCR) and ligand chain reaction (LCR). Culture is performed on Thayer-Martin plates that must be stored refrigerated but warmed to room temperature before obtaining sample. The plate is then incubated in a carbon dioxide atmosphere.

PCR and LCR are gene amplification techniques that markedly increase the sensitivity of specimen testing. Both techniques amplify the genetic fingerprint of specimens with very few organisms present in order to more easily detect and identify the organisms, PCR and LCR are not readily available because they may require a specialized lab facility.

In males Gram stain of urethral discharge show gram negative diplococcic and in females culture of cervical discharge show gram negative diplococcic.

Treatment

Non pharmacological method

- Avoid sexual contact with high-risk partners also treat infected sexual partners and use latex condoms during the intercourse.

Pharmacological method

A number of treatment options are available for the management of gonococcal infection. During earlier times, penicillins, tetracyclines, sulfonamides were widely used however due to resistance, cephalosporins and fluoroquinolones are currently used antibacteraial agents. Efficacy and safety, allergy history, age, pregnancy, patient preference and cost of the antibiotic or antibacterial agent influences the drug selection. Centers for disease control and prevention (CDC) treatment recommends following guidelines for treating non complicated gonorrhea.

- Treat gonorrhea at any anatomic site with a single intramuscular injection of 250 mg ceftriaxone and either 1gm azithromycin as a single oral dose or 100 mg doxycycline orally twice per day for 7 days.
- If ceftriaxone is unavailable, patients can be given a single oral dose of cefixime 400 gm and either a single dose of azithromycin or doxycycline 100 mg orally twice per day for 7 days.
- If the patient is allergic to cephalosporins, a single dose of azithromycin 2 gm can be used.

A cefixime dose of 400 mg is effective for urethral disease. The preferred Fluoroquinolones, ciprofloxacin, levofloxacin and ofloxacin are also highly safe and effective for treatment of uncomplicated gonorrhea but they are contraindicated during pregnancy and for children below age 18. Dissiminated gonococcal infections are best treated with a long course of intravenous ceftriaxone, cefotaxime, or ceftizoxime. Therapy should be continued for 24 to 48 hours after significant clinical improvement, (E.g., decrease in fever, and WBC count) then followed with a suitable oral agent for another 7 days.

Topical therapy with 1% silver nitrate, 1% tetracycline or 0.5% erythromycin is recommended for immediate postpartum administration to all newborns. Single dose of IM or IV ceftriaxone (25-50 mg/kg not more than 125 mg total) is recommended for treatment of gonococcal ophthalmia neonatorum and gonococcal conjunctivitis in adults.

Counseling Points

Proper education is essential to prevent gonorrhea than a simple instruction to avoid sex especially in teenaged population.

1. Recommend the use of condoms as a reasonable alternative to abstinence.
2. Patients should also be counseled about the additional risks of unprotected sex, such as the acquisition of more serious or lifelong infections such as herpes, hepatitis B and HIV, and of course, about the risks of pregnancy.
3. The emotional aspect of sexual relationships should also need to be addressed especially for teenagers who are more vulnerable for having unprotected sex.

TUBERCULOSIS

Tuberculosis is an infection caused by *Mycobacterium tuberculosis* that commonly affects lungs (pulmonary tuberculosis) and also the central nervous system (meningitis), lymphatic system, circulatory system, genitourinary system, bones and joints.

Etiology

Tuberculosis results from inhalation of airborne particles (droplet nuclei) containing *M. tuberculosis* which disperse primarily through coughing, singing, and other forced respiratory maneuvers by people who have active pulmonary TB and whose sputum contains a significant number of organisms. Droplet nuclei containing tubercle bacilli may remain suspended in room air currents for several hours, increasing the chance of spread. Individuals are at risk when they stay in over crowded, enclosed, poorly ventilated spaces. Health care practitioners who have close contact with active cases also have an increased risk.

Pathogenesis

Latent infection occurs when the tubercle bacilli are inhaled into the body. After inhalation droplet nuclei containing *M. tuberculosis* settle into the bronchioles and alveoli of the lungs. Development of infection depends upon both the virulence of the organism and inherent microbicidal ability of the alveolar Macrophages. After 14 to 21 days of infection, tubercle bacilli spread *via* the lymphatic system and blood system to other organs. The organism replicate for 2 to 12 weeks till they reach a specific number. The T cells secrete interferon-Y, interlukin-2, interlukin-10, and other cytokines and macrophages to engulf and kill the tubercle bacilli preventing further spread. At this point patient develops cell mediated immunity which can be detected by a reaction to tuberculin test.

Active Disease (Tuberculosis)

In most patients TB occurs as a result of reactivation of a previously controlled latent infection termed as reactivation tuberculosis. The apices of lungs are the most common sites for the reactivation of disease.

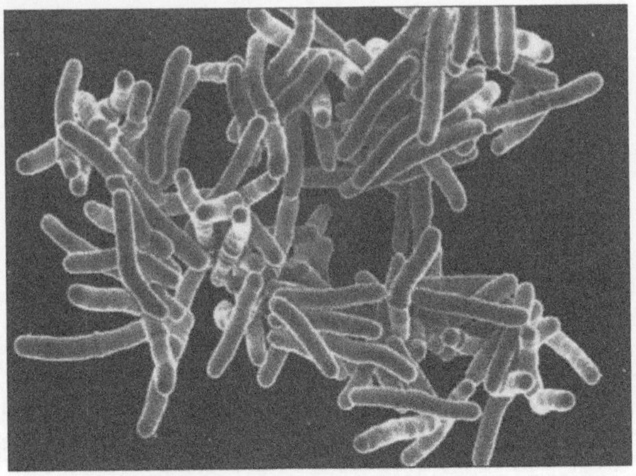

Mycobacterium Tuberculosis

Clinical Manifestations

Following are the manifestations of Pulmonary TB

- Weight loss
- Fatigue
- Productive cough
- Fever
- Night sweats
- Frank Hemoptysis

Lab Investigations

Mantoux Test: The mantoux test is the preferred TB skin test. It uses tuberculin purified protein derivative. The standard 5 tuberculin unit ppd dose is placed intracutaneously on volar aspect of forearm with a 26-27 gauge needle. The injection should produce a small raised blanched wheal. The area of induration ("bump") is the end point.

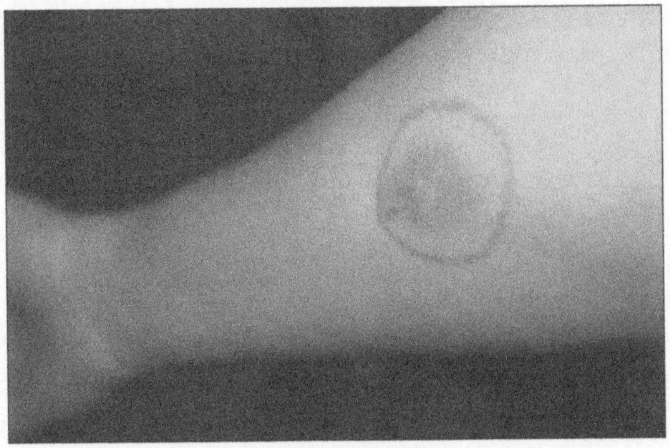

Induration

Management

Management of Tuberculosis includes both non pharmacological and pharmacological management.

Pharmacological Treatment

Objectives of pharmacological therapy are

- To kill the extracellular tubercular bacilli living in lung cavities, that are metabolically active and divide continuously.
- To sterilize and eliminate the bacilli that replicate less actively in acidic and anoxic closed lesions, and to kill semi-dormant bacilli living intracellularly in other host tissues.

Drugs Used for Treating Tuberculosis

First line drugs		Second line drugs	
Drug	**Dose**	**Drug**	**Dose**
Isoniazid (H)	5 mg/kg (Maximum recommended dose is 300 mg)	Ethionamide	15-20 mg/Kg
Rifampicin (R)	10 mg/kg (Maximum recommended dose is 300 mg)	Cycloserine	10-15 mg/Kg
Ethambutol (E)	25 mg/kg	Kanamycin	15-30 mg/Kg
Pyrazinamide (Z)	15 mg/kg	Amikacin	15 mg/Kg
Streptomycin (S)	15 mg/kg	Levofloxacin	500-1000 mg
		Ofloxacin	200 mg bid

The current treatment for the complete elimination of active and dormant bacilli involves two phases:

Initial phase: Three or more drugs (usually isoniazid, rifampicin, pyrazinamide and ethambutol or streptomycin) are used for two months, and allow a rapid killing of actively dividing bacteria, resulting in the negativization of sputum.

Continuation phase: Fewer drugs (usually isoniazid and rifampicin) are used for 4 to 7 months, aimed at killing any remaining or dormant bacilli and preventing recurrence.

Treatment Regimens

World Health Organisation prescribes the following regimens based on the category of tuberculosis:

Category	Characteristic of TB cases	Initiative phase	Continuation phase
1	New sputum smear-positive Seriously ill, sputum smear-negative Seriously ill, extra-pulmonary	2(HRZE)3	4(HR)3
2	Relapse failure treatment after default others	2(SHREZ)3 1(HREZ)3	5(HRE)3
3	Sputum smear-negative, Not seriously ill, extra-pulmonary	2(HRZ)3	4(HR)3
4	Sputum smear-negative, Not seriously ill, extra-pulmonary	Second line	

- 1, 2, 4, 5 are No. of months the treatment to be used.
- 3 is No.of days used in a week.

Counseling Points for TB Patients

Patients should be educated about the disease

- TB is a disease caused by *Mycobacterium tuberculosis* bacteria. It mainly spreads from one person to another through inhalation of air suspended droplets contaminated with Tuberculosis pathogens. The pathogen usually affects the lungs but may also cause illness in other parts of the body.
- TB is a serious illness and need combination of medications to treat the disease.
- Typical symptoms of TB are persistent cough for more than 2-3 weeks, fever for more than 7 days, shortness of breath, decrease in appetite, sudden or unexpected weight loss, fatigue, sweating at night and productive cough with sputum.

About Medication

The patients should be counseled regarding specific medications and their side effects.

Rifampicin: Rifampicin should be taken as advised by the doctor. Body fluids (tears, urine, and saliva) may turn orange colored after taking this medication. Please wear spectacles instead of soft contact lenses as they may be permanently stained.

Isoniazid: Ask patients to minimize alcohol consumption because it increases chance of hepatitis. Patient must be asked to seek medical attention if signs of liver disorder like persistent vomiting, anorexia and jaundice are developed.

Pyrazinamide: Advise the patient on how to take medication. Patient must be asked to seek medical attention if signs of liver disorder like persistent vomiting, anorexia and jaundice.

Ethambutal: Advise the patient about safe use of medication. Patient must also be told to get routine vision test done as ethambutol can cause blindness.

Besides these specific counseling points, patient must be told that medication adherence is very important and resistance to the drugs or relapse of TB may occur if medication adherence is not followed.

Recommended Lifestyle Modifications

Patient should be counseled regarding lifestyle changes as TB spreads as droplet infection.

- Patient should be asked to cover the nose and mouth with a handkerchief while sneezing or coughing.
- Patient should be advised to stay in well ventilated room where adequate sunlight and air circulation is there.
- Patient should be advised to avoid close contact with children and elderly who have weak immune system.
- Patient should be advised to dispose patient's sputum by burning or burying.

HEPATITIS

Hepatitis is defined as inflammation of the liver caused by various strains of hepatitis virus infection (e.g.: Hepatitis A, Hepatitis B, Hepatitis C, Hepatitis D and Hepatitis E), or medications (e.g.: Methyldopa or Isoniazid) or due to immunologic abnormalities (e.g.: autoimmune hepatitis). Hepatitis can occur as an acute or chronic disease. Chronic disease is generally considered as any disease or infection persisting for six months or longer. Hepatitis may be self-limiting (healing on its own) or can progress in to fibrosis (scarring) and cirrhosis. Hepatitis may occur with limited or no symptoms, but often can lead to jaundice, anorexia (poor appetite) and malaise.

According to the prognosis, Hepatitis may be classified into

Acute: Illness with discrete date of onset with jaundice or increased serum aminotransferase concentration of > 2.5 times the upper limit of normal (35-40 IV/L).

Chronic: Inflammatory condition of the liver involving an ongoing hepatocellular necrosis for 6 months or more after the onset of acute illness.

Viral hepatitis is further classified in to the following based on the type of hepatitis virus:

- Hepatitis A
- Hepatitis B
- Hepatitis C
- Hepatitis D
- Hepatitis E
- Hepatitis G

Etiopathogenesis

Viral Hepatitis

Hepatitis A: Hepatitis A infection is caused by Hepatitis A Virus (HAV) and is asymptomatic in approximately one third of the patients. It spreads through faeco-oral route and has an incubation period of 15-45 days. A month after the infection, patients typically experience the acute onset of symptoms that lasts for about 4 weeks. Patients with more severe symptoms have an increase in their serum aspartate aminotransferase (AST), alanine aminotransferase (ALT), and bilirubin, which resolve over 4 to 6 months.

Hepatitis B: Hepatitis B infection is caused by Hepatitis B Virus (HBV). It spreads through parenteral route or by intimate contact with the infected person and has an incubation period of 30-180 days. Acute hepatitis occurs in others with progression to fulminant hepatitis in less than 1%. Acute hepatitis B is typically associated with high elevations in AST and ALT (more than a 100-fold increase over normal) and bilirubin (20-fold increase over normal).

Hepatitis C: Hepatitis C infections are caused by Hepatitis C Virus (HCV). It spreads by parenteral route or by close contact and has an incubation period of 20-90 days. Serum AST, ALT and bilirubin increases in acute hepatitis C infection, but the increase tends not to be as high as in hepatitis B.

Hepatitis D: Hepatitis D infections are caused by Hepatitis D Virus (HDV). It spreads by parenteral route or by close contact and has an incubation period of 30-50 days.

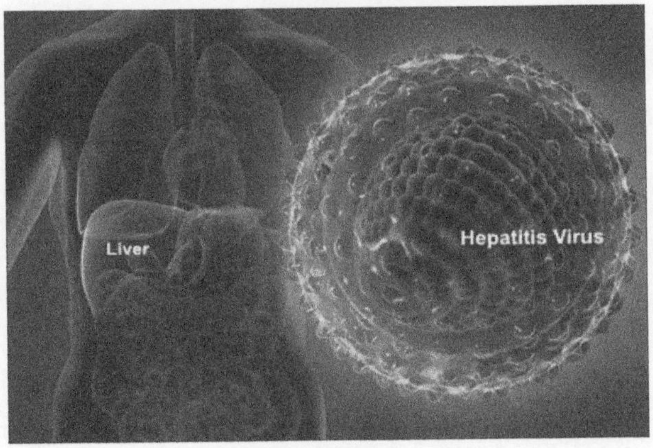

Hepatitis E: Hepatitis E infections are caused by Hepatitis E Virus (HEV). It is water-borne and has an incubation period of 20-90 days.

Hepatitis G: Hepatitis G infections are caused by Hepatitis G Virus (HGV). It spreads through percutaneous route and has an incubation period of 14-35 days.

Drug-Induced Hepatitis

Several medicines have been reported to cause liver injury as an adverse drug reaction. Drugs that cause liver injury are Amitriptyline, Amiodarone, Hormonal Contraceptives, Ibuprofen, Isoniazid, Rifampicin, Pyrazinamide, Methotrexate, Methyldopa, Phenytoin and Valproic acid.

Clinical Presentations

Viral Hepatitis

Hepatitis A is associated with the abrupt onset of symptoms, including

- Fever
- Nausea
- Anorexia
- Diarrhea
- Fatigue
- Malaise
- Abdominal discomfort
- Dark urine
- Jaundice

The severity of illness appears to be age dependent. In most cases, children have no symptoms, whereas adults usually experience symptoms and experience jaundice.

Hepatitis B and C: After the incubation period, patients who become symptomatic may develop nonspecific, flu-like symptoms such as malaise, fatigue, weakness, anorexia, nausea, vomiting, and pain in right upper part of abdomen. These symptoms start about a week before the jaundice develops. The onset of clinical symptoms is insidious and usually continues for few weeks after the development of dark urine, jaundice, and elevated serum bilirubin values.

Chronic hepatitis: The most common symptoms of chronic hepatitis are fatigue, weakness, and malaise. Some patients experience tenderness in the right upper part of the abdomen, nausea, anorexia, and muscle or joint pain. Once cirrhosis develops, the fatigue, anorexia, weight loss, and weakness become more severe. Also, patients may develop ascites, jaundice, muscle wasting, hepatic encephalopathy, and esophageal varices. A small group of patients may develop extrahepatic symptoms of chronic viral hepatitis such as arthritis and urticaria.

Drug-Induced hepatitis: The signs and symptoms of drug-induced hepatitis are highly variable and can present as acute or chronic disease. Patients may develop fever, rash, arthralgias, nausea, jaundice, abdominal complaints, lymphadenopathy, hepatomegaly, and eosinophilia. All patients have elevations in at least some liver tests (AST, ALT, alkaline phosphatase, and bilirubin). The magnitude of the elevations and the enzymes involved depend on the offending agent and the severity and stage of the liver damage.

Diagnosis

Viral Hepatitis

Hepatitis A: The diagnosis of acute hepatitis A cannot be made on clinical symptoms alone. Diagnosis is based on measurement of immunoglobulin M (IgM) antibodies to hepatitis A in the serum. Later, IgG antibodies to hepatitis A appear in the serum and protect against re-infection.

Hepatitis B: HBsAg can be measured in the serum 30 to 60 days after exposure to the hepatitis B virus. Antibodies against HBsAg develop in response to an infection with hepatitis B and provide long-term immunity. IgM antibodies against the hepatitis B core antigen also develop in response to an acute hepatitis B infection and persist for about 6 months. The IgM antibodies against the core antigen can be used as a marker for acute hepatitis B infection.

Hepatitis C: HCV infections can be diagnosed by detection of antibodies against the HCV or HCV RNA in the patient's serum. Antibodies against hepatitis C can be measured 4 to 8 weeks after infection but depends on the assay. About 15% of patients that test positive for antibodies against hepatitis C will test negative for HCV RNA.

Drug-Induced Hepatitis

The diagnosis of drug-induced liver injury requires exclusion of other causes because the symptoms of drug-induced hepatitis can be quite similar to those of hepatitis from other origins. A comparison between the time course, frequency, and type of injury the patient is exhibiting and those that have been reported is helpful in determining the likelihood that a particular reaction is drug induced.

Treatment

Non-pharmacological therapy: The development of end-stage liver disease and cirrhosis can be hastened in patients by alcohol consumption. So it is very important for patients to be counseled regarding the discontinuation of alcohol consumption.

Alternative therapies: Several clinical studies have reported positive result with silymarin (derived from the milk thistle plant) suggesting that it decreases complications and hastens recovery from hepatitis. Many studies were conducted evaluating the effects of medicinal herbs for the treatment of HCV infections. Only few agents appear to show promising results in the treatment of hepatitis C, but due to limitations in the study design it is not well known.

Pharmacotherapy

Viral Hepatitis

Hepatitis A- Pre-exposure Prophylaxis: The Center for Disease Control currently recommends hepatitis A vaccination of persons over 2 years of age, travelling to areas with increased rates of hepatitis A. The inactivated hepatitis A vaccines should be administered into the deltoid muscle. The vaccine takes about 4 weeks to induce a protective immune response and lasts for at least 20 years.

Hepatitis A- Post-exposure Prophylaxis: Immune globulin prophylaxis for hepatitis A is recommended for patients with illegal sexual contact, sharing narcotic drugs with people infected with hepatitis A. Immune globulin more than 2 weeks after exposure is not recommended.

Hepatitis B- Pre-exposure Prophylaxis: Hepatitis B vaccine series is recommended in people at high risk for exposure to hepatitis B such as infants born to infected mothers, infants/children of immigrants from areas with high rates of hepatitis B virus infection, persons sharing illegal drugs, health care and public safety workers, and patients on hemodialysis.

Hepatitis B- Post-exposure Prophylaxis: Hepatitis B immune globulin (HBIG) is produced from plasma that contains high titers of antibody against HBsAg. It is used to provide passive immunity against hepatitis B infection. Because HBIG provides only short-term protection against hepatitis B, the hepatitis B vaccine series or booster doses should also be given to these patients as appropriate. HBIG (0.06 m*l*/kg for adults and children) should be administered through IM injection, preferably into the deltoid muscle or the antero lateral aspect of the thigh as soon after exposure to the hepatitis B virus.

The hepatitis B vaccine is a recombinant product in which common baker's yeast is used to produce a noninfectious subunit of HBsAg. The series of three IM injections (second and third doses are given 1 and 6 months, respectively, after the first dose) produces an adequate antibody response in adults and children. The deltoid muscle is the recommended location for injection for adults and children because injections into the buttocks produce a lower response rate. The anterolateral thigh muscle should be used for infants and neonates.

Chronic Hepatitis B

Interferon was the first approved agent used to treat chronic hepatitis B. Several types of in terferons are commercially available like interferon α-2a and α-2b, interferon α-n3, interferon alfacon-1, interferon β-1a and β-1b, and interferon γ-1b. Interferon has antiviral and immune stimulatory properties and may be beneficial in treating viral hepatitis. Interferon α-2b at a dose of 5 million international units (IU) subcutaneously daily or 10 million IU three times weekly for 16 weeks for HBeAg-positive patients and 12 months for HBeAg-negative patients has been used to treat chronic hepatitis B infection with some success. Interferon treatment is associated with flu-like symptoms (fever, fatigue, headache, and myalgia) in some patients. Administering interferon at bedtime improves tolerability to this drug. Some patients also have photosensitivity reactions while on interferon and should be encouraged to use sunscreen and protective clothing.

Lamivudine, an antiviral drug, is an irreversible inhibitor of reverse transcriptase that blocks hepatitis B viral replication. Chronic hepatitis B treatment in HBeAg-positive patients with lamivudine 100 mg daily per oral results in loss of HBeAg, normalization of ALT and histologic improvement. Greatest concern with lamivudine use is high incidence of hepatitis B viral mutation and drug resistance. The most common adverse effects with lamivudine are headache, malaise, fatigue, nausea, vomiting, diarrhea, neuropathy, cough, congestion, and musculoskeletal pain. Dose adjustments must be made for patients with renal insufficiency.

Adefovir is an acyclic nucleotide analogue with antiviral activity against hepatitis B. In HBeAg-positive and HBeAg-negative patients, Adefovir 10 mg daily is used in the treatment of chronic hepatitis B. The most common adverse effects associated with adefovir are nausea, diarrhea, vomiting, dyspepsia, headache, and weakness. Pruritis and rash have also been reported.

Entecavir is a guanosine nucleoside analog with selective activity against hepatitis B virus. Entecavir has been approved by FDA at a dose of 0.5 mg orally once a day or in lamivudine-resistant patients at a dose of 1 mg orally once a day.

Hepatitis C

For those patients who have not previously been treated for hepatitis C and have chronic hepatitis C genotype 1, peginterferon (α-2a or α-2b) plus ribavirin 1,000 to 1,200 mg per day result in sustained viral response (SVR) and is superior to conventional interferon plus ribavirin treatment. For patients with genotypes 2 or 3, interferon (conventional or pegylated) plus a lower dose of ribavirin at 800 mg per day may result in sustained viral response in most of the patients. Ribavirin is highly teratogenic and embryotoxic, and therefore should not be used in women who are pregnant or in men whose female partners are pregnant. Major side effects of combination treatment include flu like symptoms (headache, fever, fatigue, myalgia, nausea), hematologic side effects (anemia, leukopenia, thrombocytopenia), and depression.

Drug-Induced Hepatitis

The most important step that can be taken in a suspected clinically significant drug-induced liver injury is discontinuation of the offending agent. Management of the liver injury should be supportive.

Patient Counseling in Hepatitis

- ***Knowledge about the disease and transmission:*** Patient must be provided information about Hepatitis disease and also made aware of strategies to be implemented to reduce its transmission to others.
- ***Fluid intake:*** Plenty of fluid must be taken by the patients as less intake of fluid may lead to dehydration.
- ***Diet:*** Avoid taking fatty and oil rich diet as digestion is improper during the disease condition. Also avoid intake of protein rich diet as it may lead to accumulation of proteins which may lead to complications like hepatic encephalopathy.
- ***Alcohol consumption:*** The development of end-stage liver disease and cirrhosis can be hastened in patients by ethanol consumption. Thus it is very important to counsel patients about discontinuation of alcohol consumption.
- ***Risk reduction plans:*** Risk Reduction Plans are the tools to initiate discussions with patients about risk behaviors and are sample of strategies that may reduce the risk. Avoiding Injecting Drug Use (IDU), illegal sexual contacts, tattooing/body piercing, and alcohol reduction are the risk reduction strategies to prevent the exposure to infection.

Avoidance of hepatotoxic and nephrotoxic drugs

- Hepatotoxic dugs like acetaminophen should be avoided as it may cause liver toxicity and also the drugs used for the treatment of hepatitis like anti viral drugs must be used with caution in patients with kidney damage as they may lead to nephrotoxicity.

LEPROSY

Leprosy is a chronic infectious disease caused by acid-fast, rod-shaped bacteria called as *Mycobacterium leprae* that primarily affects the skin, the peripheral nerves, the mucosa of the upper respiratory tract, and the eyes. Leprosy may lead to progressive damage of these structures and results in disfigurement and disability permanently. Leprosy was known to exist since 4000 BC and the disease was described in the ancient civilizations of China, India, and Egypt. The first known written reference to the disease on Egyptian papyrus dates from about 1550 BC. Leprosy affects the individuals of all ages. The signs and symptoms of leprosy are visible lately from several weeks to 20 years or more due to slow multiplication of the organism. Apart from human beings, other animals such as armadillos, chimpanzees, and mangabey monkeys serve as reservoirs of infection. Leprosy is thought to be transmitted *via* droplets from the nose and mouth during close prolonged contact with affected individuals. Due to immunological protection, only 5-10% of the infected individuals develop the signs and symptoms of Leprosy.

Signs and Symptoms

Signs and symptoms of leprosy vary based on the immune response of an individual to *M leprae*. The WHO classifies leprosy in to Paucibacillary (PB) and Multibacillary (MB) leprosy based on the number of skin lesions and nerve involvement. However, within the WHO's simplified classification, there can be a fairly wide range of patient presentations.

- Paucibacillary leprosy

  (Two to five skin lesions with negative skin smear results at all sites)
- Paucibacillary single lesion leprosy

  (One skin lesion with negative skin smear results at all sites)
- Multibacillary leprosy

  (Six or more skin lesions or positive skin smear results at any site)

The Ridley-Jopling classifies leprosy further into five different categories based on the severity of the disease such as Tuberculoid leprosy, Borderline tuberculoid leprosy, Mid-borderline leprosy, Borderline lepromatous leprosy, and Lepromatous leprosy.

Following are the common signs and symptoms of leprosy and vary with the form of the disease.

(a) Flat or raised reddish or copper colored skin lesions or nodules.

(b) Single or multiple skin lesions found on face, buttocks, and extremities

(c) Thickening of the skin and peripheral nerves and leading to loss of sensation

(d) Ulcerations of the skin

(e) Peripheral nerve involvement leading to muscle weakness

(f) Testicular involvement leading to sexual dysfunction or sterility

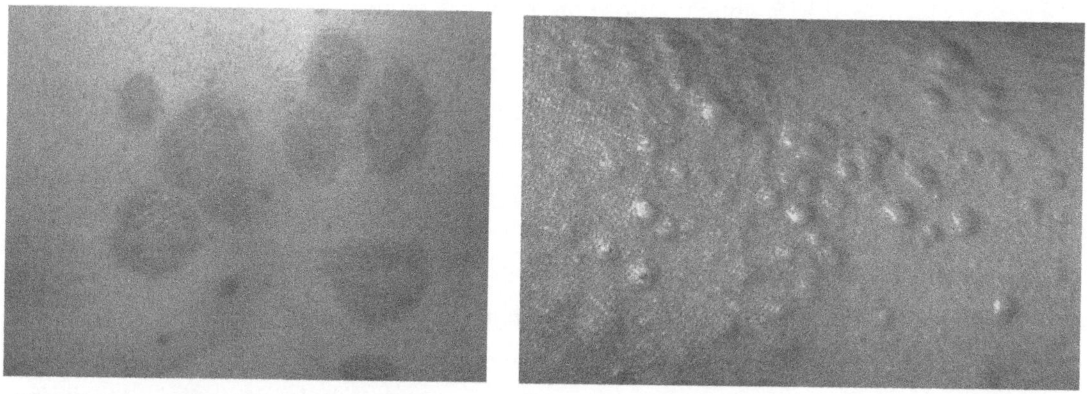

Fig. 11.1 Erythematous Maculae, with Little Desquamation, Disseminated in the Trunk

(a) Eye involvement including eye pain, eye redness, inability to close the eyelids, corneal ulcers, and blindness
(b) Loss of eyebrows and eyelashes
(c) Destruction of the nasal cartilage

Diagnosis

Diagnosis of leprosy is often established from the patient's clinical signs and symptoms, laboratory examinations include skin smears or skin biopsies. Ziehl-Neelsen stain or the Fite stain is used to diagnose leprosy. Other less commonly used tests include blood exams, nasal smears, and nerve biopsies.

Leprosy Management

Patients should be educated to inspect their hands and feet for possible injuries sustained and that may go unnoticed due to loss of sensation. Prescribed medications stand primary for successful treatment of leprosy. Compliance with full course of medications is vital in successful management. Ulcers or tissue damage can result, leading to skin infections and disability. Thus proper foot wear and injury prevention should be encouraged.

Pharmacotherapy

World Health Organization (WHO) recommends multidrug therapy with three medications for the management of Leprosy. They are a) Dapsone, b) Rifampicin and c) Clofazimine. WHO distributes the medications in convenient monthly calendar blister packs to patients at free of cost. After taking the first doses of these medications, patients will not transmit the disease to others. Resistance of *M. leprae* to MDT has not developed yet. WHO currently recommends different treatment regimens for patients with paucibacillary leprosy and multibacillary leprosy.

WHO Recommendations for Leprosy Management

Paucibacillary single-lesion leprosy

- A single dose of Rifampicin, Ofloxacin or Minocycline,
- Six months of treatment with Rifampicin (monthly) and Dapsone
  1. Paucibacillary leprosy
  2. Multibacillary leprosy
- Twelve months of treatment using Rifampicin (monthly), Dapsone, and Clofazimine

U.S. Recommendations

Paucibacillary leprosy

- Twelve months of treatment using rifampicin (daily) and dapsone

  Multibacillary leprosy
- Twenty-four months of treatment using rifampicin (daily), dapsone, and clofazimine

  Individuals who develop type 1 or type 2 reactions may require other medications.

Type 1 reaction (reversal reaction): Treatment may include the use of corticosteroids, salicylates, and nonsteroidal anti-inflammatory drugs (NSAIDs).

Type 2 reaction (ENL): Treatment may include the use of Corticosteroids, salicylates, NSAIDs, clofazimine, and thalidomide

Surgical Therapy

There are various surgical procedures available to certain patients with leprosy. These surgical procedures are aimed at restoring function of affected body parts, cosmetically improving areas damaged by the disease, amputation of affected body parts, drain a nerve abscess or to relieve the compression of nerves.

Follow-up

Patients should maintain close contact with their health-care provider during treatment with MDT, and periodic follow-up visits are recommended. The WHO recommends the monthly direct supervision by a health-care provider during the administration of Rifampicin. Periodic blood testing during treatment is recommended, as well as yearly skin scrapings when possible. The relapse rate after the administration of MDT is about 1%. Therefore, patients should still be followed by a health-care provider for five to 10 years after completion of MDT. Some patients with leprosy may require psychological counseling, physical therapy, and occupational therapy.

Leprosy Prevention

The prevention of leprosy ultimately lies in the early diagnosis and treatment of those individuals suspected or diagnosed as having leprosy. This strategy prevents further transmission of the disease to others. Public education and community awareness campaigns encourage individuals with leprosy and their families to undergo evaluation and treatment with MDT. Household contacts of patients with leprosy should be monitored closely for the development of leprosy signs and symptoms. A recent study demonstrated that prophylaxis with a single dose of rifampicin was 57% effective in preventing leprosy for the first two years in individuals who have close contact with newly diagnosed patients with leprosy. Currently, there is no single commercial vaccine that confers complete immunity against leprosy in individuals. In certain populations, some vaccines, including the BCG vaccine, provide variable levels of protection against leprosy.

SUGGESTED READINGS

1. 2008 European guidelines for the management of syphilis. [Online]. 2008 Dec 1. [Cited on 2011 Feb 1]; Available from URL: http://www.ncbi.nlm.nih.gov/pubmed/19386965
2. Background document: The diagnosis, treatment and prevention of typhoid fever. World Health Organization. [Online]. 2003 May. [Cited on 2011 Feb 1]. Available from URL: http://whqlibdoc.who.int/hq/2003/WHO_V&B_03.07.pdf
3. Kasper DL, Braunwald E, Fauci AS, Hauser SL, Longo DL, Jameson JL, editors (2005). Harrison's principles of internal medicine. 16th ed. New York: McGraw Hill medical publishing division.

4. Kasper DL, Braunwald E, Fauci AS, Hauser SL, Longo DL, Jameson JL, editors (2005). Harrison's principles of internal medicine. 16th ed. New York: McGraw Hill medical publishing division.

5. Koda Kimble Mary Anne, Young Lloyd Yee, Alldredge Brian K, Corelli Robin L, Guglielmo B. Joseph, Kradjan Wayne A, Williams Bradley R (2009). Applied Therapeutics: The Clinical Use Of Drugs, 9th Edition. Lippincott Williams & Wilkins.

6. Public health notifiable disease management guidelines- Amoebiasis, Alberta Health and wellness, Canada [Online]. 2005 October. [Cited 2011 Feb 1]. Available from the URL: http://www.health.alberta.ca/documents/ND-Amoebiasis.pdf

7. Ratnam S. (2005). The laboratory diagnosis of syphilis. *Can J Infect Dis Med Microbiol*; **16(1):** 45-51.

8. Sexually transmitted diseases- Syphilis. Centres for disease control and prevention. [Online]. [Cited 2011 Feb 1]Available from URL: http://www.cdc.gov/std/syphilis/default.htm

9. Singh S. 2001. Symposium-Typhoid fever, pathogenesis and laboratory diagnosis. Indian Academy of Clinical Medicine **2(1):**17-20.

10. Standard Treatment Guidelines- Amoebiasis. Ministry of Health & Family Welfare, Government of India. [Online] [Cited 2011 Feb 1]. Available from the URL: http://www.mohfw.nic.in

11. Walker R, Whittlesea C, editors. (2008) Clinical pharmacy and therapeutics, 4th ed. Edinburgh: Churchill livingstone-Elsevier.

CHAPTER 12

RESPONDING TO SYMPTOMS OF MINOR AILMENTS

LEARNING OBJECTIVES

- Know the definition of the ailment
- Understand the pathophysiology and symptoms
- Know the non pharmacological and pharmacological management strategies

PAIN

Introduction

Pain is an unpleasant, subjective sensory and emotional experience associated with the actual or potential tissue damage. As per the American Academy of Pain Medicine, pain is defined as "An unpleasant sensation and emotional response to that sensation". Dr. Don Ranney, in his book **"Anatomy of Pain"** defines pain as – "A perception, not really a sensation, in the same way that vision and hearing are. It involves sensitivity to chemical changes in the tissues and then interpretation of such changes as harmful. This perception is real, whether or not harm has occurred or is occurring. Cognition is involved in the pain perception. Pain may be generated by noxious peripheral stimuli or by lesions within the peripheral and central nervous systems.

Types of Pain

Pains are broadly classified in to

(i) Nociceptive pain and

(ii) Neuropathic pain.

(i) Nociceptive pain arise from the stimulation of superficial or deep tissue receptors (nociceptors) E.g., Pain associated with conditions like burns, fractures of bone, appendicitis, surgical procedures or myocardial ischemia.

(ii) Neuropathic pain arises from a disturbance of neural pathways at any point from the primary afferent conducting system to receptive centers in the central nervous system

(CNS). This is due to nerve cell or axonal cell dysfunction due to compression, E.g., diabetic neuropathy and nerve plexus avulsion. The pain resulted due to a primary lesion in the CNS; such pain is called as neuropathic pain.

Pathophysiology

Damage to the tissue by mechanical, thermal or chemical means directly excites peripheral nerve endings on the nerve membranes. This causes the release of chemical mediators such as potassium and hydrogen ions, serotonin, bradykinin, substance P, thromboxanes, leukotrienes, nerve growth factors and histamines. Release of the inflammatory mediators sensitizes primary afferent nociceptor neurons resulting in inflammation, pain and sensitivity in the injured area.

Excitation of primary afferent nociceptors release number of neurotransmitters at the spinal cord synapses. The excitatory neurotransmitters (Glutamate and Aspartate) mediate fast nociceptive transmission by acting at N- Methyl D-Aspartate (NMDA) receptors. As a result, there will be an increased production of diffusible neurotransmitter Nitric oxide, which acts to increase release of glutamate, enhancing nociceptive transmission and contributes to central sensitization. Activated phospholipase A_2 enzyme increases arachidonic acid.

CENTRAL PATHWAYS

Several ascending pathways in the spinal cord (spinothalamic, spinoreticular and spinomesencephalic) tracts transmit nociceptive information from the dorsal horn to the supraspinal sites in the brain stem, thalamus and cortex.

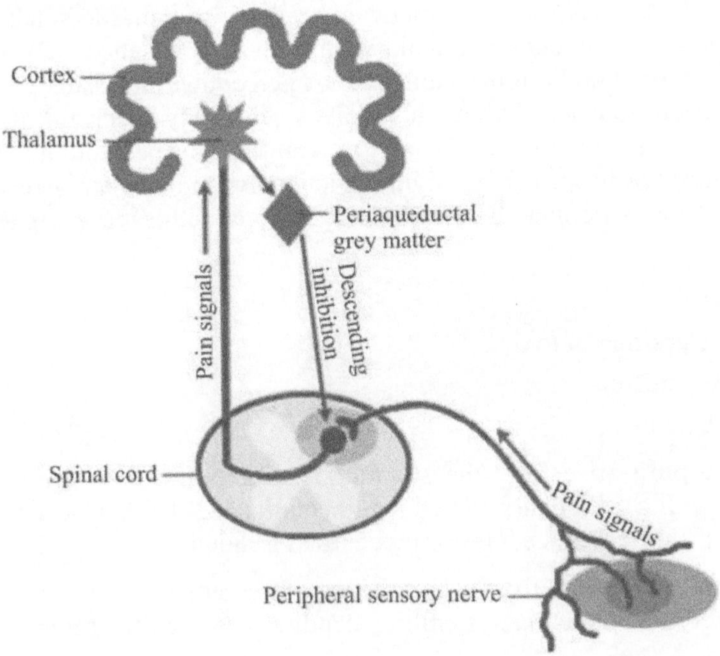

CLINICAL PRESENTATIONS

Symptoms: Pain can be described as sharp, dull, burning, shock like, tingling, shooting, radiating, fluctuating in intensity and varying in location. Nonspecific symptoms include anxiety, depression, fatigue, insomnia, anger and fear.

Acute pain may cause hypertension, tachycardia, diaphoresis, mydriasis and pallor. However these signs are not diagnostic. In some acute cases and chronic cases no obvious signs are present. Pain is always subjective; thus pain can be best diagnosed based on patient's description and history.

Nociceptive pain is often acute, localized, well described and relieve with conventional analgesics. Neuropathic pain is often chronic, not well described and not easily treated with conventional analgesics.

Management of Pain

Acute Pain

- ***Non Steroidal Antiinflammatory Agents:*** Non Steroidal Anti Inflammatory Agents block the prostaglandins produced by arachidonic acid cascade, thereby decreasing the number of pain impulses received by the CNS.

E.g.,	Acetylsalicylic acid	-	325-650 mg every 4 hours
	Paracetamol	-	650 mg every 6 hours
	Ibuprofen	-	400 mg every 8 hours

- ***Opioid Agents:*** Opioid agents include the following classes of drugs like

  Morphine and their agonists: Morphine, Hydromorphone, Oxymorphone

  Meperidine and their agonists: Meperidine and Fentanyl

  Methadone and their agonists: Methadone and Propoxyphene

  Morphine agonists-antagonists derivatives: Pentazocine, Butorphanol, Nalbuphine

  Opioid antagonist: Nalaxone

- ***Central Analgesics:*** Tramadol

Morphine and congeners are considered to be the first line drugs for moderate to severe pain. It can be given as oral, parenteral or rectal. Nausea and vomiting are more likely with the initial dose in ambulatory patients. Respiratory depression increases progressively as doses are increased. Respiratory depression can be reversed by Nalaxone.

Meperidine and congeners are less potent and has a shorter duration of action than Morphine. With high doses or in patients with renal failure, the metabolite Normeperidine accumulates causing tremors, muscle twitching and possibly seizures.

Methadone and congeners has oral efficacy, extended duration of action and ability to suppress withdrawal symptoms in heroine addicts. But it results in excessive sedation. It is usually used for chronic pain.

Opioid agonist-antagonist derivatives produce analgesia and have a ceiling effect on respiratory depression and lower abuse potential than morphine.

Opioid antagonists: Nalaxone is a pure opioid antagonist that binds completely to opioid receptors but does not produce analgesic response. It is used to reverse the toxic effects of Opioids in the dose of 0.4 to 2.0 mg through I.V/I.M/subcutaneous routes.

Central analgesic: Tramadol binds to μ receptors that inhibit the opiate receptors and weakly inhibits serotonin and norepinephrine reuptake. Thereby Tramadol produces the pain relief. Tramadol is used in the dose of 50 mg to 100 mg in moderate to severe pain relief. It is mainly used in the treatment of neuropathic pain. Side effects may include risk of seizures.

CHRONIC PAIN

Non steroidal anti inflammatory drugs (NSAIDS) are effective for skeletal muscle pains. **Methadone** can be used for treating cancer pain since it has prolonged mechanism of action. Epidural clonidine is also effective for treatment of refractory pain. Tricyclic antidepressants and anticonvulsants are also used for the relief of neuropathic pain.

Non-pharmacological techniques

Physical techniques considered as nonpharmacological measures include physiotherapy, hyper stimulation analgesia, muscle relaxation, biofeedback, nerve blocks, and surgery.

Psychological techniques practiced to alleviate the pain are assertiveness, behavioral modification, counseling, hypnosis, psychotherapy, stress management, art and music therapy. Social techinques include the community support groups, occupational therapy, and self-help groups.

ROLE OF THE PHARMACIST IN PAIN MANAGEMENT

Pain is an unpleasant or an inconvenience experience. Pain contributes to adverse clinical, economic, and personal outcomes. Pain lowers satisfaction with care and interferes with functioning. Pain is an important element in morbidity, mortality. Majority patients with chronic clinical conditions suffer from the pain. About 85% of the post operative patients complain the symptoms of pain. Pain medications such as NSAIDs and Opioid analgesics may relieve the pain sensations however they have serious tendency for abuse, misuse, diversion, and addiction. In such situation, community pharmacists have tremendous opportunities to analyze the drug therapy, assess drug related issues and advice patients on suitable pain management.

CASE STUDY

Mrs. NK, a 30 year old bank employee visited your pharmacy and asked for pain relief medication for her severe headache. She mentioned that, she experiences the headache more often at weekends. Mrs. NK has asked you for a suitable medication and advice.

Information Collection and Processing

Headache is a subjective symptom. There are several different types of headaches. Based on the symptoms, headaches are classified in to tension headache, migraine headache, cluster head ache, and ice pick head ache. Mrs. NK should be asked to describe the symptoms to assess the type of head ache. As Mrs. NK has a severe throbbing headache with nausea and photophobia, it sounds as Migraine type of headache. In this situation, Mrs. NK's may be recommended with Paracetamol 650 mg for three times a day and Mrs. NK should be referred to a Neurologist for further evaluation and treatment.

Nausea and Vomiting

Nausea and vomiting are the most commonly seen complaints in patients suffering from gastro intestinal disorders and chronic conditions like cancer. Nausea is a symptom, which is subjective and an unpleasant sensation of urge to vomit. It is followed by variety of autonomic signs such as pallor, sweating, tachycardia, salivation and increased respiratory rate. Vomiting or emesis is the reflex expulsion of the stomach contents via the esophagus and mouth and is usually associated with nausea and retching. Retching is an involuntary but unsuccessful effort to vomit.

Etiology

Nausea and vomiting are experienced in various clinical situations like gastrointestinal tract obstruction, mucosal lesions such as ulcers, inflammation, liver diseases, pancreatic and small intestinal diseases, peritonitis, cardiovascular disease such as myocardial infarction, renal failures, diabetic ketoacidosis, hyperparathyroidism, adrenal insufficiency, pregnancy and gynecologic disorders such as pelvic inflammation and complications of pregnancy, neurological disorders such as increased cranial pressure, hemorrhage, epilepsy, meningitis, migraine, vertigo, meniere's syndrome, brain metastases, psychiatric disorders, drug withdrawal syndrome, radiation therapy, operative procedures and acute gastroenteritis, ingestion of certain obnoxious substances, ingestion of certain drugs like opiates, general anesthetics, and antineoplastic agents.

Clinical Presentation

The signs and symptoms of vomiting include dehydration, weight loss, mental confusion, reduced skin turgor, increased thrust, hypotension, muscle weakness or cardiac rhythm disturbances, and alkalosis.

Pathophysiology

There are three consecutive phases of emesis:

- Nausea
- Retching
- Vomiting

Nausea is an urge to vomit and is associated with gastric stasis and may be considered as a separate and singular symptom.

Retching is the labored movement of abdominal and thoracic muscles before vomiting.

The final phase of emesis is **Vomiting**, the forceful expulsion of gastric contents caused by GI retro peristalsis.

The pathophysiology involved in vomiting is mainly mediated via the stimulation of the vomiting centre. The afferent fibers from the sensory receptors in the pharynx, stomach, intestine and other visceral organs connect directly to the vomiting centre through the vagus and splanchnic nerve and stimulate the vomiting centre.

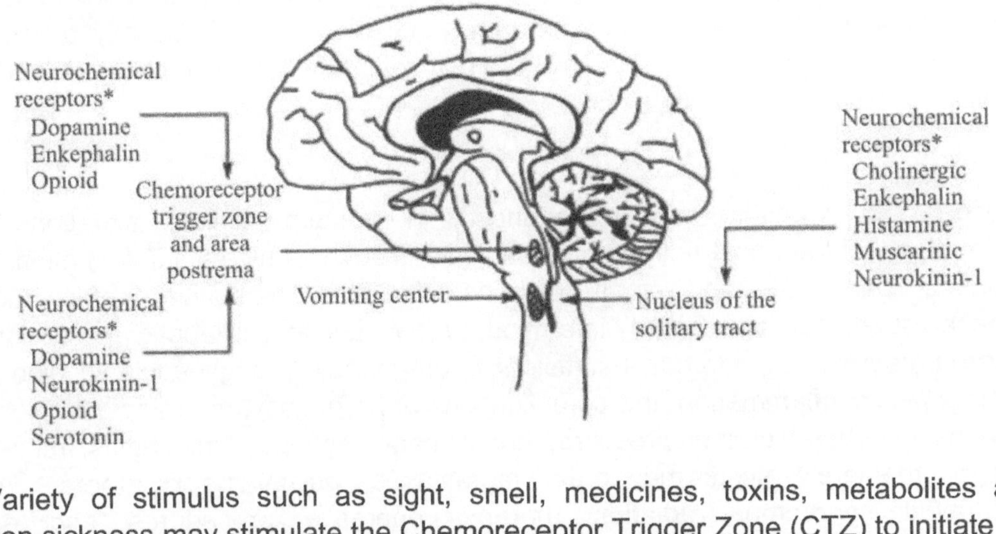

Variety of stimulus such as sight, smell, medicines, toxins, metabolites and motion sickness may stimulate the Chemoreceptor Trigger Zone (CTZ) to initiate the vomiting reflex. When the vomiting centre is stimulated, the efferent impulses are sent to the salivary, vasomotor and respiratory centers. Five major neurochemical transmitter systems are involved in causing vomiting. These receptors are present in the vomiting centre and the chemo trigger zone. When they receive the stimulus they act via their respective receptors to produce emesis.

The main neurotransmitters involved in producing vomiting are:

- Dopaminergic
- Histaminic
- 5-hydroxytryptamine 3
- Cholinergic
- Substance P

The dopaminergic receptors are present in the CTZ and GI tract. The dopamine agonists like apomorphine and levodopa are thought to mediate vomiting via this pathway. Whereas in motion sickness there is an imbalance in the cholinergic and adrenergic system in the region of the medulla near vomiting center and CTZ or directly stimulate the CTZ. The chemotherapeutic agents produce nausea and vomiting through serotonin stimulating the receptor located on afferent vagal nerve terminals to initiate vomiting reflex. Substance P- a neuropeptide that belongs to tachykinin family is found in high concentration in the nucleus tractus solitaries and the area postrema of CNS. The actions of substance P are mediated through NK1 receptor.

PROCESS OF VOMITING

Vomiting reflex begins with a sudden deep inspiration that increases the abdominal pressure. This pressure is further increased by the contraction of the abdominal muscles. Further the soft palate rises and the epiglottis closes, preventing the aspiration of vomitus into the lungs. In the next step, the pyloric sphincter and the esophagus relax and allowing the stomach contents to be expelled out and flow of saliva increases to aid the expulsion.

Management of Nausea and Vomiting: Management of Nausea and Vomiting includes both non pharmacological and pharmacological methods.

Non-pharmacological Management: It includes a variety of dietary, physical or psychological changes. Ex: For patients with simple complaints resulting from excessive food or disagreeable foods, moderation or avoidance is preferable. Behavior modification and guided mental imagery also identified as non-pharmacological methods but efficacy of these techniques is yet to be established.

Pharmacological Management

Medications used in the management of nausea and vomiting are classified as:

1. *Antacids and antisecretory agents:* Antacids act locally in the stomach by neutralizing gastric acid and can be used to relieve nausea and vomiting related to

gastric acid or heartburn. E.g., Magnesium and Aluminum hydroxide containing tablets or suspensions.

2. ***Histamine 2-receptor antagonists:*** E.g., Cimetidine, Famotidine, Nizatidine, and Ranitidine.
3. ***Proton pump inhibitors:*** Proton pump inhibitors are helpful in managing nausea and vomiting related to excess gastric acid secretion. E.g., Omeprazole, Esomeprazole, Lansoprazole, Pantoprazole, and Rabeprazole.
4. ***Anticholinergics:*** Anticholinergic agent Scopolamine blocks muscarinic receptors in the vestibular system, thereby block signals to the central nervous system (CNS). It is effective for preventing and treating motion sickness and preventing post operative nausea and vomiting as well. E.g., Scopolamine: 0.5 mg every 72 hours.
5. ***Antihistamines:*** Antihistamines are commonly used to prevent and treat nausea and vomiting due to motion sickness, vertigo, or migraine headache. Their efficacy is presumably due to the high concentration of histamine (H_1) and muscarinic, cholinergic receptors within the vestibular system. Undesired effects include drowsiness and blurred vision. E.g., Diphenhydramine: 10-150 mg every 4-6 hours as needed.
6. ***Dopamine antagonists:*** Stimulation of dopamine D_2 receptors in the CTZ leads to vomiting. Phenothiazine anti-emetics act via inhibiting the dopaminergic action in the CTZ. They can be used in severe motion sickness, vertigo, migraine, gastritis etc. they cause sedation, orthostatic hypotension and extra pyramidal side effects such as dystonia. E.g., **Chlorpromazine**: 10-25 mg Q 4-6 hr, **Promethazine**: 12.5-25 mg Q 4-6 hr as needed. **Domperidone** is a D_2 receptor blocker and prevents the nausea and vomiting. It is used in the dose of 10 mg 8th hourly.
7. ***Serotonin antagonists***: Release of 5-HT leads to stimulation of visceral vagal nerve fibers and CTZ, thereby causing vomiting. Selective 5-HT_3 receptor antagonist inhibits the release of 5-HT, thereby prevent vomiting. They are used to treat chemotherapy induced vomiting and post operative nausea and vomiting. E.g., Ondansetron: 32 mg IV prior to chemotherapy as single dose or 1.5 mg /kg prior to chemotherapy, repeat every 4-8 hours or 8 mg orally prior to chemotherapy, repeat at 4 & 8 hours every 12 hours for 1-2 after completion of chemotherapy.

Nausea and vomiting is an inconvenience to the individual. The cause of the nausea and vomiting should be evaluated before initiating the treatment. In the following conditions, patient should be referred to doctor immediately.

- Poisoning is suspected.
- The patient has been vomiting for longer than 24 hours.
- There is blood in the vomit.
- The patient complains of severe abdominal pain or headache and stiff neck.
- There are signs of dehydration such as dry mouth, infrequent
- Urination or dark urine

CASE STUDY

Mr. SR a 25 year old salesman approached you in your pharmacy and complains of nausea which he is experiencing since 2 days after taking food in a local restaurant. Next day onwards he was experiencing the sensation. He is also feeling like his stomach is filled with gas (Bloating). He is currently not on any medication.

Mr. SR's presentations suggest that gastritis induced nausea. Since he had food in a restaurant, it might be was spicy and irritating the GI. His presentations include nausea and bloating. Excess secretion of acid stimulates the CTZ in the CNS and causes nauseating feeling. Acidity also produces gas in the stomach and makes the person feel full in the stomach. In order to overcome the problem Mr. SR may be advised to take Ranitidine 150 mg and Domperidone 10 mg bid for three days and to chew Gelusil MPS an antacid tablet t.i.d to neutralize the excess acid and Methyl Poly Siloxane (MPS) to clear the bloating. Mr. SR should be advised to take bland diet for next few days till symptoms completely clear. If no progress in condition is observed, he may be advised to consult the doctor for further evaluation.

DYSPEPSIA

The term 'dyspepsia' is derived from Greek word. The meaning of Dyspepsia is "improper digestion" and is used to describe upper abdominal discomfort, usually related to food or alcohol intake or certain medications like antibiotics, non steroidal anti inflammatory drugs (NSAID), digoxin, bisphosphonates, theophylline. Smoking and stressful lifestyle may also contribute to the development of dyspepsia.

Chronic dyspepsia is defined as recurrent symptoms that include epigastric pain, abdominal bloating, belching, nausea, vomiting and early satiety. The four major causes of investigated dyspepsia include peptic ulcer disease, gastro esophageal reflux disease with or without esophagitis, malignancy and functional or idiopathic dyspepsia. The term 'functional' indicates that function is abnormal but there is no identified mucosal damage or cause and is often resistant to treatment.

Pathophysiology

Several pathophysiologic mechanisms are involved in the development of functional dyspepsia, including visceral hypersensitivity, both in the stomach and the duodenum, impaired gastric accommodation, antral over distention, delayed gastric emptying, and abnormal duodeno jejunal motility. Acute infrequent dyspepsia is commonly associated with irregular intake of food, regular intake of alcohol, cigarette smoking, and stress. Chronic dyspepsia is related to peptic ulcer disease, esophageal reflux disease, H pylori infection, and malignancy. Irritable bowel syndrome may also contribute to functional dyspepsia.

Clinical Features

Acute infrequent dyspepsia is self limiting and generally requires no further investigation. But symptoms like concomitant weight loss, persistent vomiting, constant severe pain, dysphasia, hematoemesis, or melena warrants endoscopy. Patients with functional dyspepsia are often younger and present variety of abdominal and extra gastrointestinal complaints, show signs of anxiety or depression. Alarming symptoms include early satiety, anorexia, worsening dysphagia, unexplained weight loss (> 10 % of body weight), vomiting, anemia, GI Bleeding, jaundice, and history of PUD.

The clinical assessment of uninvestigated dyspepsia in patients with age < 55 years with no alarming symptoms can be identified through H Pylori test. Recent onset of dyspepsia in an older individual may be considered as an independent factor to develop underlying malignancy such as gastric cancer. Dyspeptic patients older than 55 years with or without alarming symptoms should undergo upper GI endoscopy.

MANAGEMENT OF DYSPEPSIA

Non-pharmacological Therapy

Lifestyle modifications like bland diet, smoking cessation, reduced intake of alcohol and weight reduction through aerobics are the right strategies to prevent this condition. Symptoms will improve in patients who practice altered lifestyle modifications, discontinue the alcohol consumption and reduced intake of caffeine and fatty foods.

PHARMACOLOGICAL THERAPY

Antacids

Mixtures of aluminum and magnesium salts are appropriate combination to prevent the bowel upsets. Antacids cause mucosal protection by neutralizing the acid and forming a coat on damaged tissue. Suspensions are more effective than the tablets but are less convenient for patients with frequent symptoms. Antacids should be taken regularly in a dose of 15 ml t.i.d for effective relief of symptoms.

H_2 Receptor Antagonists

H_2 receptor antagonists such as Ranitidine, Famotidine, blocks the action of histamine on H_2 receptors of the parietal cells thus reducing the basal and stimulated gastric acid secretion. Due to good therapeutic efficacy Famotidine 20 mg BID or 40 mg OD and Ranitidine in 150 mg BID or 300 mg OD are effective in providing relief in dyspepsia.

Antisecretory Agents

Proton pump inhibitor (PPIs) binds irreversibly to the $Na^+ K^+$ ATPase pump and inhibits the terminal step in the acid production. PPIs inhibit both basal and stimulated gastric acid secretions. Proton Pump Inhibitors are more effective when taken 30-60 minutes before the first meal on an empty stomach. Proton pump inhibitors like Omeprazole 20 mg OD, Rabeprazole 20 mg, Lansoprazole 30 mg OD, Pantaprozole 40 mg are commonly used PPIs in the management of Dyspepsia.

SUCRALFATE

Sucralfate is an aluminium salt of a sulfated disacchride protects gastric mucosa by shielding ulcerated tissues from acid, pepsin and bile salts. Sucralfate binds to the ulcerated mucosa at pH 2.0-2.5 and protects the mucosa by forming a barrier on mucosa. Sucralfate in the dose of 1 gm QID or 2 gm BID is indicated to reduce the symptoms of dyspepsia.

Other Pharmacological Agents

The prokinetic agent Metoclopramide at dose of 5-10 mg three times daily is found useful in improving the symptoms. However it should be used only on medical advice due to its neuropsychiatric side effects. This agent enhances the release of gastric acetylcholine through dual inhibition of D_2 receptors and acetylcholinesterase. Further, evaluation of H pylori presence through breath urease test and giving eradication medications benefit the patients from symptoms of dyspepsia.

Alternative Therapies

Herbal therapies using peppermint, caraway may benefit some patients with symptoms of dyspepsia.

ROLE OF COMMUNITY PHARMACIST IN THE MANAGEMENT OF DYSPEPSIA

Pharmacist has a great role in managing the symptoms of dyspepsia. Community pharmacist may enquire the patients about their food habits, social history and life style habits. If the patient is having any risk factors such as cigarette smoking, alcohol consumption, stressful life events, OTC medication usage etc., he or she may be educated about them. For symptomatic relief, patient may be advised to take antacids or H_2 blockers and may be dispensed as OTC. However the pharmacist should encourage the patient to see the doctor immediately.

CASE STUDY

Mr. UK, a 35 year old sales executive presents at the pharmacy counter and asking for Gelusil MPS for his heart burn. Upon enquiry he explains that he often gets heart burn especially after he eats at a restaurant, where his favorite meal is fried chicken and chips which he takes once in a week. He also told that, recently he is experiencing more heartburn after any large meal, especially at night when he goes to bed. When he was asked to describe the pain, he says it is burning and it rises up, and he points to his upper chest, around the sternum area. He has used Gelusil MPS and as he felt a relief he wants to continue to use the same. Mr. UK is well built and little overweight. When you have asked him about any other medication he is using, he tells that he has been prescribed an anti-inflammatory for his ankle pain, which he got hurt whilst playing football a few weeks ago. He takes the anti inflammatory drug every day. He is also taking Doxy-1 for his acne every night and he also takes alcohol during the social outings.

Effective counseling involves three steps

1. Information gathering
2. Information processing
3. Information delivery

Information Gathering

Background Information

Heartburn

Heartburn is also called as gastro esophageal reflux disease (GERD). It is estimated that 15-20% of the adults experience heartburn once a week. Many individuals will experience the symptoms after dietary indiscretion or excessive alcohol consumption. Some individuals experience potentially life threatening disorders such as deep ulceration, intractable stricturing, malignancy arising in columnar metaplasia (Barrett's esophagus) as GERD complications.

For patients with alarming symptoms, therapy should be given for few weeks. If symptoms improve, the treatment may be continued. If symptoms are not subsided, or patient has alarming symptoms such as pain in swallowing, dysphasia, weight loss or anemia, the patient should be referred to a consultant for further evaluation.

Appropriate medications should be used for the relief of symptoms. Life style modifications such as brisk walking, avoidance of alcohol and large meals and smoking cessation should be practiced. Where possible, patients should be encouraged to stop medications known to cause GERD (e.g., NSAIDs, Calcium channel blockers and Theophylline).

Information required from Mr. UK.

Information regarding his problem may be collected by asking following questions.

- Please describe your symptoms
- Since how long you have these symptoms?
- What makes these symptoms better or worse?
- How effective is Gelusil MPS for you?
- How often do you take Gelusil MPS?
- Describe your diet?
- What other medications are you taking?
- When and how do you take diclofenac tablets?

Information Processing

Gathered information should be processed for suitability of the treatment, any other drug related problems and to provide appropriate information.

Based on the information given by Mr. UK, it may be noted that, Mr UK is taking Diclofenac sodium for his ankle injury and Doxycycline for his acne. He is also taking spicy food that may aggravate disease condition.

In GERD conditions, use of Diclofenac Sodium may further aggravate the GERD condition. In such situations, simple analgesic like Paracetamol may be used if little or no inflammation is present.

Doxycycline may commonly cause epigastric burning and esophagitis. It should be taken with a glass of water and the patient should remain upright for at least half an hour after administration.

The effect of Doxycycline may moderately decrease if antacid is taken together with Doxycycline. Mr. UK's diet is also equally important in reducing the symptoms.

Information delivery

The following points should be discussed with Mr.UK.

Appropriate dosing of Doxy-1 to help minimize adverse effects

- Take Doxy-1 with food and wash down with a full glass of water.
- Remain up right for at least 30 minutes after taking the tablet.
- Avoid excessive sun exposure as this can cause photosensitivity reactions.

Advice on Diclofenac usage

Mr. UK should be informed to take diclofenac tablet with food to minimize the gastric irritation.

Advice on GERD

- Avoid excessive alcohol and smoking
- Avoid large meals
- Reduce your body weight
- See the doctor for further evaluation and advice.

Appropriate treatment for sprains and strains

- If feasible, stop using Diclofenac and take Paracetamol.
- Remind Mr. UK that the best management for sprains and strains at the time of injury is rest, ice, compression and elevation (RICE)

DIARRHEA

Diarrhoea is defined as an increase in frequency and fluidity of stool. Normally a healthy human individual defecate about 200 gm of stool per day. But during diarrhea, more than 250 gm stool containing 70-95% water will be produced and the frequency is increased up to 5-20 times/day. In severe cases, more than 1.4 L of fluid may be lost. During diarrhea, an individual may experience a self limited minor discomfort accompanied by pain and urgency. Dysentery is called as a low volume, painful and bloody diarrhea. The morbidity and mortality with diarrhea is largely attributed to dehydration.

Diarrhea may occur due to ingestion of contaminated food or water with virus, bacteria, or protozoal pathogens. Common causative bacterial organisms are Shigella, Salmonella, Vibrio, Campylobacter, Staphylococcus and Escherichia coli and viral infections with Norovirus and Rotavirus. Other causes for diarrhea are poor personal hygiene, travel history, compromised immune status, medications such as antibiotics, antacids containing magnesium, NSAIDs, prostaglandins etc. Surgical reduction of gut length, neural dysfunction, irritable bowel syndrome, hyperthyroidism, diabetic neuropathy, carcinoid syndrome are responsible for causing diarrhea.

World Health Organisation (WHO) classifies diarrhea in to

- ***Acute diarrhea*** - commonly defined as the diarrhea with less than 14 days' duration (e.g., Infectious diarrhea)
- ***Chronic diarrhea*** – Diarrhea with more than 14 days' of duration.

PATHOPHYSIOLOGY

Diarrhea occurs due to an imbalance between absorption and secretion of water and electrolytes. It may be associated with a specific disease of the intestine or secondary to a disease outside the intestine.

The principal mechanisms of diarrhea are

- Change in the active ion transport by either a decreased sodium absorption or an increased chloride secretion.
- Change in the intestinal motility.
- Increase in luminal osmolarity.
- Increase in tissue hydrostatic pressure.
- Malabsorption.

Types of Diarrhea

Based on the pathophysiologic mechanisms, diarrhea may be classified in to

1. ***Secretory diarrhea***: It occurs due to mucosal epithelium damage caused by a stimulating agent such as pathogenic toxins (Bacterial and Viral origin), vasoactive intestinal peptide (5-HT and prostaglandins). These substances may increase the

secretion or decrease the absorption of water and electrolytes. In Secretory diarrhea an output of more than 500 mL of stool per day will be produced.

2. ***Osmotic diarrhea***: It is caused by the retention of poorly absorbed substances in the intestinal lumen which exert excessive osmotic forces leading to the output of more than 500 mL of stool per day, which abates upon fasting. Osmotic diarrhea can occur due to Disaccharidase (lactase) deficiencies, Lactulose therapy (for hepatic encephalopathy, constipation), Magnesium containing antacids.
3. ***Exudative diarrhea:*** Inflammatory diseases of the gastrointestinal tract cause exudative diarrhea by the discharge of mucus, proteins or blood into the gut. This may be caused by mucosal epithelium damage by bacterial infections (Shigella, Entamoeba, and Salmonella), or idiopathic inflammatory bowel disease. This leads to an output of purulent and bloody stools that persist even on fasting. Stools are frequent and may be of small or large volume.
4. ***Malabsorption:*** Improper absorption of gut nutrients produces voluminous, bulky stools with increased osmolarity combined with excess fat (steatorrhea). This type of diarrhea usually decreases with fasting.

MANAGEMENT

Prevention of excessive water and electrolyte loss are the main strategies in the management of diarrhea. Both non pharmacological and pharmacological management eliminates the causes and provide symptom relief.

Non-pharmacological Management

Non pharmacological strategies to prevent the symptoms of diarrhea include eating bland diet and avoiding solid foods and dairy products at least for 24 hours. In replenishing the lost electrolytes, oral rehydration salts (ORS) may be recommended. Many commercial formulations are available as ORS. An ORS meeting the WHO formula is more appropriate to be given. Formulas containing excess electrolytes may cause nausea and vomiting. ORS formula can also be made at home by mixing a pinch of salt in to 200 mL of boiled and cooled water with one tea spoonful of sugar.

Pharmacological Management

Various classes of drugs are used to treat diarrhea such as to antimotility, adsorbents, antisecretory compounds, antibiotics, enzymes and drugs that increase intestinal micro flora.

Anti-motility drugs: These drugs delay the transit of intra luminal content or increase the gut capacity, prolonging contact and absorption.

E.g., Loperamide – Generally used in acute and chronic diarrhea.

Adult dose: Initially 4 mg then 2 mg after each loose stool but should not exceed 16 mg/day.

Diphenoxylate – 5 mg four times daily but do not exceed 20 mg/day.

Opiates and opioid derivatives – Opium tincture may be given as 0.6 ml four times daily but Opium tincture is having addiction potential.

Adsorbents: Adsorbents are used to provide symptomatic relief. These are non-specific in action and act by adsorbing nutrients, toxins, drugs and digestive juices. Co-administration with other drugs reduces their bioavailability.

E.g., Kaolin-pectin – Given at a dosage range of 30-120 mL after each loose stool.

Antisecretory Agents

Antisecretory agents are often used to treat traveler's diarrhea. E.g., Bismuth subsalicylate. Adverse effects include darkening of the tongue and stools, tinnitus and encephalopathy at high doses.

Bacterial replacement agents: Lactobacillus preparations (Lactobacillus acidophilus, Lactobacillus bulgaricus) are intended to replace the colonic microflora, thereby restoring the intestinal function and suppressing the growth of pathogenic microorganisms.

Dose: 2 tablets or 1 granule packet with milk, juice or water is given 3-4 times in a day.

Octreotide: It is a synthetic octapeptide analog of endogenous somatostatin. It is given of the symptomatic treatment of carcinoid tumors and vasoactive peptide (VIP) secreting tumors. It acts by blocking the release of serotonin and other active peptides and thus controls diarrhea and flushing. The dosage range for managing diarrhea associated with carcinoid tumors is 100-600 mcg/day in 2 or 4 divided doses subcutaneously. The adverse effects include nausea, abdominal pain, choleliathiasis and diarrhea.

ANTIBACTERIAL AGENTS

Antibacterial agents are used to kill the responsible pathogens such as Escherichia coli, Campylobacter, Shigella, Salmonella causing mucosal damage of the epithelium and causing bloody diarrhea. These agents include antiameobic agents such as Enteroquinol, metronidazole and tinidazole formulations, and antibiotics such as Flouroquinolones eg: Norfloxacin 400 mg or Ciprofloxacin 500 mg or Oflaxacin 200 mg. Combinations of Flouroquinolones and antiameobic agents are also used to control infective bloody diarrheas.

CASE STUDY

Mr. NG a 43 year old vegetable vendor visited the pharmacy and asked for a tablet to control his loose stools. Upon enquiry he presented the symptoms of increased frequency (5 times) of his stools which is watery in consistency with cramps in the stomach, foul smelling with passing gas.

Mr. NG revealed that he had taken chat food items at a road side stall. Next day he had a feeling of nausea and bloating initially and later he had five times watery diarrhea. He did not have any food since morning and he is feeling slightly sick.

The main reason for his symptoms may be the protozoa infected food. Mr. NG presentations have a similarity with the symptoms of amebic dysentery. Thus he may be asked to see the doctor for further evaluation. He may be advised to take drink Oral Rehydration Salts (ORS) or tender coconut to replenish the water and electrolytes. Further he may be dispensed with

Tablet. Ranitidine 150 mg with Domperidone 10 mg bid

Tablet. Metronidazole 400 mg tid for 5 days.

Amoebic dysentery is protozoal infections which occur due to consumption of infected food. Often this occurs in individuals who eat food unhygienly prepared. The symptoms include frequent loose stools with mucus and foul smelling, fever, abdominal cramps, hyperacidity and bloating.

Ranitidine is a H_2 blocker that blocks the H_2 receptor mediated hyper secretion of acid. Domperodone helps in preventing the nausea and vomiting associated with CTZ stimulation. Metronidazole is an antiprotozoal and kill amoeba and there control the infection.

To clear the symptoms of hyperacidity induced bloating Mr. NG may be advised to chew Tab. Gelusil MPS t.i.d after food.

Mr. NG may be recommended to and eat food of bland in nature once symptoms come in to control and also advised not to eat food sold at roadside.

CONSTIPATION

Constipation is defined as an infrequent bowel action of twice a week or less that involves straining to pass hard stools accompanied by a sensation of pain or incomplete evacuation. Constipation appears to be more common in up to 20% in elderly people, 8% of middle – aged and 3% of young people. Poor diet, insufficient intake of fluids, lack of exercise, concurrent disease states and use of multiple drugs are the predisposing factors to constipation.

Constipation is not a disease but is a symptom of an underlying disease or problem. Diseases or conditions that may cause constipation are:

A. Gastrointestinal disorders

- Gastro duodenal obstruction from ulceration or cancer, irritable bowel syndrome, diverticulitis, haemorrhoids, anal fissures, ulcerative proctitis, tumors

B. Metabolic and endocrine disorders

- Diabetes mellitus, Hypothyroidism, Panhypopituitarism, Pheochromocytoma, Hypocalcaemia

C. Pregnancy

D. Neurogenic constipation

- Head trauma, Central nervous system tumors, Stroke, Parkinsons disease

E. Psychogenic constipation

- Psychiatric disorders. Inappropriate bowel habits

PATHOPHYSIOLOGY

The gastrointestinal tract is divided in to upper and lower gastrointestinal tracts. The upper gastrointestinal intestinal tract is responsible for ingestion and digestion of the food where as the lower gastrointestinal tract is responsible for conserving body water and electrolytes, drying the feces and elimination. The remains of undigested food are swept along the GI tract through "peristalsis" the waves of muscular contractions. These peristaltic waves eventually move the faeces from the colon to the rectum and induce the urge to defecate. By the time stool reaches the rectum it become more solid in consistency because most of the water has been absorbed. Normally there is a net uptake of fluid in the intestine in response to osmotic gradients involving the absorption and secretion of ions, absorption of sugars and amino acids. This process is under the influence of autonomic nervous system. In some situations where absorption increases will generally lead to constipation. Agents that alter intestinal motility either directly or by acting on the autonomic nervous system affect the transit time of food. A slower transit time will lead to the formation of hard stools and constipation. Motility is largely under parasympathetic control, with stimulation bringing about an increase in motility while antagonistic such as anticholinergics, or drugs with anticholinergic side effects, decrease motility and induce constipation. Opioids induce constipation by other mechanism. They cause constipation by maintaining or increasing the tone of smooth muscle, suppress forward peristalsis, raise sphincter tone at the ileocaecal valve and anal sphincter and reduce sensitivity to rectal distension. This delays the passage of faeces through the gut with a resultant increase in absorption of electrolytes and water in the small intestine and colon.

Management

General measures to manage the constipation include dietary modification (increase in the amount of fiber content daily) exercise, change in bowel habits to urge for defecate, and increasing fluid intake. If an underlying disease is recognized as the cause of constipation, attempts should be made to correct the disease. Gastro Intestinal malignancies may be removed through a surgical resection. Appropriate methods should be used to correct endocrine and metabolic derangements. It is important to assess the potential drug causes for constipation and take suitable strategies to resolve the same.

Non-pharmacological Treatment

Non pharmacological treatment includes:

- Increased intake of water up to 2 liters
- Avoidance of excess intake of coffee or tea.
- Consuming foods that contain more fiber such as fruits, vegetables, and cereals.
- An increased level of exercise

Pharmacologic Therapy

Three types of laxatives are commonly used in the management of constipation.

1. Those causing softening of feces in 1 to 3 days e.g., Bulk-forming laxatives, Docusates, and lactulose
2. Those result in soft or semi fluid stool in 6 to 12 hours e.g., bisacodyl and senna
3. Those causing water evacuation in 1 to 6 hours e.g., saline cathartics, castor oil, and Polyethylene glycol-electrolyte lavage solution

Bulk-forming agents in addition to dietary fiber intake will improve the condition.

For most non-hospitalized persons with acute constipation, the infrequent use of most laxative products is acceptable. For example, acute constipation may be relieved by the use of a tap-water enema or a glycerine suppository. If neither is effective, use of oral sorbitol, low doses of bisacodyl or senna, or saline laxatives (e.g., milk of magnesia) may provide relief.

If laxative treatment is required for longer than 1 week, the person should be advised to consult a physician to determine underlying causes for constipation that requires treatment with agents other than laxatives.

For some bedridden or geriatric patients, or others with chronic constipation, bulk-forming laxatives remain the first line of treatment, but the use of more potent laxatives may be required relatively frequently. Agents that may be used in these situations include milk of magnesia and lactulose.

In the hospitalized patient without any GI disease, constipation may result due to the use of general anesthesia and/or opiate substances. Most orally or rectally administered laxatives are recommended. E.g., a tap-water enema or glycerine suppository or milk of magnesia.

Emollient Laxatives (Docusates)

These surfactant agents, docusates in its various salts, work by facilitating the mixing of aqueous and fatty materials within the intestinal tract. They may increase water and electrolyte secretion in the small and large bowel. These products result in a softening of stools within 1 to 3 days. Emollient laxatives are not effective in treating constipation but are used mainly to prevent constipation. They may be helpful in situations where straining at stool should be avoided, such as after recovery from myocardial infarction, with acute perianal disease, or after rectal surgery.

Lubricants

Mineral oil is the only lubricant laxative in routine use and acts by coating stool and allowing easier passage. It decreases colonic absorption of water, thereby increasing stool weight and reducing stool transit time. Generally, the effect on bowel function is noted after 2 or 3 days of use.

Lactulose and Sorbitol

Lactulose is a disaccharide that causes an osmotic effect retained in the colon. It is generally not recommended as a first-line agent for the treatment of constipation because it is costly and not necessarily more effective than agents such as milk of magnesia. It may be justified as an alternative for acute constipation and has been found to be particularly useful in elderly patients. Occasionally, the use of lactulose may result in flatulence, cramps, diarrhea, and electrolyte imbalances. Thus Sorbitol, a monosaccharide, has been recommended as a primary agent in the treatment of functional constipation in cognitively intact patients. It is as effective as lactulose and also economical.

Saline Cathartics

Saline cathartics are composed of relatively poorly absorbed ions such as magnesium, sulfate, phosphate, and citrate, which produce their effects primarily by osmotic action to retain fluid in the GI tract. These agents may be given orally or rectally. A bowel movement may result within few hours of oral doses and in 1 hour or less after rectal administration. These agents should be used primarily for acute evacuation of the bowel, which may be necessary before diagnostic examinations, after poisonings, and in conjunction with some antihelminthetic drugs to eliminate parasites. Agents such as milk of magnesia (8% suspension of magnesium hydroxide) may be used occasionally (every few weeks) to treat constipation in otherwise healthy adults. Saline cathartics should not be used on a routine basis to treat constipation.

Castor Oil

Castor oil is metabolized in the GI tract to an active compound, ricinoleic acid, which stimulates secretory processes, decreases glucose absorption and promotes intestinal motility, primarily in the small intestine resulting in bowel movement within 1 to 3 hours of administration. It should not be used for routine treatment of constipation as it possesses strong purgative action.

Glycerin

This agent is usually administered as a 3-g suppository and exerts its effect by osmotic action in the rectum. As with most agents given as suppositories, the onset of action is usually less than 30 minutes. **Glycerin** is considered as safe laxative although it may occasionally cause rectal irritation. Its use is acceptable on an intermittent basis for constipation, particularly in children.

Other Agents

Tap-water enemas may be used to treat simple constipation. The administration of 200 mL of water by enema to an adult often results in a bowel movement within 1.5 hours.

PYREXIA

The word Pyrexia is derived from the Greek 'pyretos' meaning 'fire'. Pyrogen is a substance that induces fever. These can be either internal (endogenous) or external (exogenous).

Exogenous pyrogens are derived from outside the patient; most of them are microbial products, microbial toxins, or whole microorganisms. Example of an exogenous pyrogen is the lipopolysaccharide produced by all gram-negative bacteria. Pyrogenic products of gram-positive organisms include the enterotoxins of Staphylococcus aureus.

Endogenous pyrogens are cytokines, molecules that are a part of the innate immune system. They are produced by phagocytic cells. Major endogenous pyrogens are interleukin 1 (α and β), interleukin 6 (IL-6) and tumor necrosis factor-alpha.

Pyrexia

Pyrexia is defined as a condition when the body temperature of an individual rises above the normal range of 36-37 °C (98-100 °F), Fever is the temporary increase in the body's temperature in response to some disease or illness. The body temperature can be measured by inserting thermometer in oral cavity, axillary, rectum and tympanic membrane of the body.

Types of Fevers

Fever may be classified in to

Continuous Fever: If the temperature remains above normal for long period of time is called as continuous fever. e.g., fever in lobar pneumonia, typhoid, and urinary tract infection.

Intermittent Fever: If the type of fever wherein the body temperature periodically rises and falls. e.g., malaria.

Relapsing Fever: Fever type that recurs several days after the temperature has returned to normal, e.g., infective endocarditis.

Signs and symptoms of Fever:

- Shivering
- Anorexia
- Dehydration
- Lethargy
- Poor concentration
- Sleepiness
- Cold

During high fevers, there may be an extreme irritability, confusion, delirium and convulsions.

Medications that Increases the Body Temperature

1. Antimicrobials E.g., Isoniazid
2. Anti-arrhythmia Drugs E.g., Procainamide, Quinidine
3. Anti-epileptic Drugs E.g., Phenytoin, Carbamazepine
4. Anti-hypertensive Drugs, E.g., Alpha-methyldopa
5. Anti-fungal Drugs, E.g., Amphotericin B
6. Ephedrine
7. Sulfa Drugs
8. Interferons
9. Narcotics/Illicit Drugs, E.g., Cocaine,Cannabis

MANAGEMENT

Non-pharmacological Methods

Majority people do not require specific treatment to cure the fever. In general, people are advised to keep adequately hydrated using oral rehydration salts and water. Tepid sponging is recommended if the body temperature rises to the level of hyperpyrexia.

Prevention

Fevers are commonly caused by bacterial/viral infections. Good hygiene practices will reduce the risk of developing an infection. Hand washing before and after meals, and after using the wash rooms is a good practice to prevent the infections. Infected people should be cared suitably to prevent further spread of the infection and care giving individuals are also advised to take suitable precautions.

During the Course of Fever

(i) If the fever is mild, drink plenty of fluids and take rest.

(ii) Remove excess clothing or blankets. The room should be comfortable, not too hot or cool. Try one layer of lightweight clothing, and one lightweight blanket for sleep. If the room is hot or stuffy, a fan may help.

(iii) A lukewarm bath or sponge bath may help in cooling someone with fever. This is especially effective after medication is given. Do NOT use cold baths, ice, or alcohol rubs. These cool the skin, but often make the situation worse by causing shivering, which raises the core body temperature.

Home Remedies to Cure the Fever

(a) Bed rest

(b) If the fever is high, apply cold compresses on the forehead, and sponge the whole body with tepid water. You can add a few drops of lavender leaves or gentle soothing perfume to the water used. This takes away the sour smell of fever.

(c) Fevers caused by gastro-intestinal problems and respiratory infections respond well to a teaspoonful of turmeric powder added to a glass of hot milk with sugar to taste.

(d) Mint: Take a handful of crushed fresh mint leaves, 2-3 black peppercorns, 2-3 long peppers, a one-fourth-inch piece of ginger, and ground to a fine paste. Boil it in two cups of water. Once it comes to the boil, simmer it for 12-15 minutes. The cooled, filtered mixture, divided into three doses and sipped as herbal tea gives relief in fevers associated with gastro-intestinal disorders.

(e) Lemon-grass tea, with honey to taste, is a refreshing remedy for fever.

In high fever, the application of cool sandalwood paste on the forehead brings the temperature down just like a cold compress does.

Pharmacological Management

To reduce the fevers, Paracetamol 325 to 650 mg 6th hourly is recommended for individuals aged more than 12 years. For children in the age group of 4-11 years, the recommended dose is 320-500 mg 6th hourly. For less than 4 years of age, the recommended dose is 5 ml (16 mg/ml).

Role of Pharmacist in the Management of Fever

For an immediate relief, pharmacist may dispense suitable dose of Paracetamol to the patient for 2-3 doses. If the fever is still persisting, patient should be advised to consult the doctor for further evaluation and management. Further patients may be advised about the non pharmacological measures to control the fever related symptoms. Some people take the paracetamol regularly for analgesics purpose. Such individuals should be advised to seek the medical opinion regarding their head ache or any other related problems. Excess intake of paracetamol in alcoholics may damage the liver. Such individuals should be cautioned about the paracetamol use.

CASE STUDY

Mr. GK a provision stores owner has visited your pharmacy and told that, he is feeling a raised body temperature since morning and asked for suitable remedy.

Information Collection and Processing

Upon enquiry, Mr. GK told that, he was experiencing the feeling of raised body temperature since morning after he started attending to his work. On physical examination, Mr. GK was found to have increased body temperature. His body temperature was found 101 °F. Mr. GK was advised to take paracetamol 650 mg thrice daily and asked to take bed rest and drink plenty of water.

Next day upon enquiry, Mr. GK told that he is feeling better. His fever has come down.

In Mr. GK's case, he experienced the fever may be due to work stress. The symptoms were resolved upon taking suitable bed rest and taking paracetamol. Paracetamol is being the safe antipyretic, people may be safely advised to take the paracetamol in this kind of situations. In case if fever does not subside probably Mr. GK should be advised to see the doctor.

OPHTHALMIC SYMPTOMS

Red Eye (Conjunctivitis)

Red eye is a minor subconjunctival hemorrhage to more severe chemical burn, most often it is called as conjunctivitis and commonly referred as 'pink eye'. Common causes for conjunctivitis include blepharitis, corneal abrasion, foreign body, keratitis, iritis, glaucoma, and scleritis. In addition to the redness, patients may experience eye discharge, pain, photophobia, itching, and visual changes. There are certain distinctive signs that assist in identifying the cause of red eye, such as watering and itching.

Allergic Conjunctivitis

Allergic conjunctivitis is usually a bilateral condition caused by pollen or other allergens. In cases where only one eye comes into contact with the allergen, the response may be unilateral. Typical symptoms of allergic conjunctivitis include red, itchy eyes associated with tearing and burning that gradually disappear when the patient is no longer in proximity to the allergen responsible. The condition is often associated with runny nose, itching of the soft palate of the mouth and sneezing. Approximately 70% of patients with allergic conjunctivitis also have asthma and/or atopic dermatitis.

Cold compresses and tear substitutes are useful in relieving burning and dry eyes in patients with a mild allergy. However, many patients require more aggressive therapy with selective histamine-1 (H_1)-receptor antihistamines (e.g., levocabastine) that relieve itching and watery eyes. Ketotifen (available as OTC) is a multiple-action H_1-receptor antihistamine that prevents the activation of inflammatory mediators. The first- and second-generation oral antihistamines are effective in treating allergic conjunctivitis and topical ophthalmic products are superior in treating this condition.

For rapid but short-lived relief of redness, patients may choose a topical decongestant such as naphazoline, tetrahydrozoline, or oxymetazoline. These are available as single-ingredient OTC preparations, including All Clear, Murine, and Visine, respectively. Preparations such as Naphcon-A, Opcon-A, and Visine-A are combinations of a topical decongestant and an antihistamine. When recommending topical decongestants, it is important to note that these products can cause further complications such as conjunctivitis and irritation if used over long periods of time. If OTC medications do not provide effective relief within 7 days or the condition worsens, patients should be referred to the ophthalmologist for further investigation. Prescription medications for allergic conjunctivitis include mast-cell stabilizing agents such as sodium cromolyn and nedocromil, as well as anti-inflammatory agents and topical nonsteroidal anti-inflammatory drugs (NSAIDs), such as ketorolac.

Bacterial Conjunctivitis

Acute bacterial conjunctivitis is characterized by a copious, purulent discharge, mild-to-moderate pain with a tingling sensation, and diminished vision. Other symptoms include red eye with a foreign body sensation. The best diagnostic indicator is glued eye(s) upon waking. Bacterial conjunctivitis can only be treated using prescription medications; therefore, patients should be referred to their physician.

Blepharitis

Chronic inflammation of the eyelids causes a condition known as blepharitis. Patients commonly complain of an itchy, gritty, uncomfortable red eye that is worse upon waking. It is not uncommon to see dandrufflike scaling on eyelashes, missing or misdirected eyelashes, and swollen eyelids. Patients should be advised that they should wash the eyelids with diluted baby shampoo or eye scrub solution. Gentle lid massages and warm compresses will also provide some relief. If patients experience relief within a month, this treatment may be continued indefinitely. If this fails, however, a prescription ophthalmic antibiotic may be required. Oral antibiotics and topical steroids may be required in severe cases.

Episcleritis

The episclera is the layer found under the conjunctiva, covering the white of the eye. Inflammation of this layer presents as redness as a result of dilation of the blood vessels that are found in this layer. This maybe sectoral whereby only one part is affected or diffuse in which case most of the episclera is inflamed. Episcleritis is commonly self-limiting and resolves itself within 3 weeks. In rare cases, episcleritis has been associated with rheumatoid arthritis. Patients with recurring episodes should be referred to an ophthalmologist. Topical NSAIDs and topical steroids may be prescribed for severe cases.

Herpes Simplex

Herpes simplex is a viral infection that first appears between the age of 6 months and 5 years. The herpes simplex virus-1 strain affects the eyelids, conjunctiva, and cornea. Typically, the patient presents with an uncomfortable eye, pain, redness, tearing, photophobia, and blurred vision. It is not uncommon to see herpetic vesicles on the eyelids or skin around the eye that rupture, crust, and heal without scarring after about 7 days. All patients presenting with a herpes simplex eye infection should be referred to their physician or ophthalmologist.

Antiviral treatment using topical or oral agents is the mainstay of therapy. Topical trifluridine 1% solution (administered 5-8 times per day) and 200 to 400 mg of oral acyclovir administered 5 times daily are available by prescription. Other options include acyclovir ophthalmic ointment, oral valacyclovir (500 mg 2-3 times daily) and oral famciclovir

(250 mg twice daily). Since topical antivirals can cause toxicity if used for more than 2 weeks they are generally avoided. Similarly, topical steroids are not recommended since they can worsen the infection.

Marginal Keratitis

Marginal keratitis is an inflammation of the cornea characterized by reduced vision, a painful red eye, sensitivity to light, foreign body sensation, and a mucopurulent discharge. It is a common, transient, usually unilateral condition that may be associated with chronic staphylococcal blepharitis. Patients presenting with the above listed symptoms should be referred to an ophthalmologist for a diagnosis. Marginal keratitis can be successfully treated using topical steroids.

Subconjunctival Hemorrhage

A subconjunctival hemorrhage is characterized by red, flat discoloration due to bleeding from the small blood vessels that run through the conjunctiva. The most common cause for spontaneous subconjunctival hemorrhage is idiopathic in nature. The condition is painless, clearing itself within 7 to 14 days. In few cases, the redness may be associated with bleeding disorders, the use of anticoagulants, conjunctivitis, scleritis, or trauma to the eye. Warm compresses may be useful in symptomatic relief. Treatment involves the identification and appropriate management of the underlying cause.

Uveitis

Uveitis or iritis is an inflammation of the iris, the ciliary body, or the choroid. Iritis may result in pain that radiates to the brow and temple; it develops with time along with redness in the eye. Other symptoms of iritis include watering, red eye, blurred vision, and photophobia. Iritis should be referred for further investigation. Patients are commonly treated with steroid eye drops to alleviate the pain and inflammation.

Arcus Senilis

Arcus senilis (corneal arcus) is a bilateral condition manifesting as a white ring in the periphery of the cornea. It is a lipid-rich corneal deposit that does not affect the patient's vision. It begins at the top and bottom of the cornea and spreads to form a complete ring. It is most commonly seen in elderly patients. Therefore, arcus senilis in patients below 50 years of age should be referred for a lipid profile, since it may indicate hyperlipidemia, hypercholesterolemia, or hyperlipoproteinemia. However, the relationship between arcus senilis and cardiovascular disease is yet to be established.

Dry Eye Syndrome

Dry eye syndrome, due to decreased production of tears or excessive tear evaporation, causes discomfort and soreness. Patients may also complain about a foreign body sensation in the eye(s). Underlying causes of dry eye include Sjögren's syndrome, aging, staring at a computer screen for too long, blinking problems, and environmental factors. Additionally, patients taking such medications as oral contraceptives, antihistamines, and beta-blockers may experience dry eyes. Pharmacists are in an ideal position to discover this adverse reaction.

Dry eye syndrome can be managed using nonprescription artificial tear products (e.g., Murine Tears Dry Eyes, Visine Tears Dry Eye Relief). Many OTC products are available, and preservative-free formulations are recommended if the patient experiences itching and irritation with the drops (e.g., Bion Tears, Refresh Celluvisc). Dryness can also be prevented by the use of humidifiers. Cyclosporine eye drops that increase tear production are available by prescription (e.g., Restasis).

Floaters

Patients describe floaters as dark specks or cobwebs that are seen in the field of vision. They are shadows of the fibers that clump together in the vitreous gel. While floaters are a normal part of the aging process and occur as some point or another in most patients, individuals suddenly experiencing new floaters, with or without flashing lights, should be referred to an ophthalmologist immediately.

Nevus

A pigmented or nonpigmented mole on the conjunctiva of the eye is known as a nevus. The nevus may be flat or slightly raised. Since nevus is normally harmless, no treatment is necessary, unless they become malignant. Patients should be referred for further investigation if the nevus is growing. The presence of nevus on the iris is an indication of neurofibromatosis type 1, an autoimmune disease.

Styes

A bacterial infection of the eyelash follicle causes a painful swelling at the margin of the eyelid known as a stye. The causative organism is usually Staphylococcus species. Warm compresses are typically recommended to provide symptomatic relief and quicken recovery. In most cases the stye will heal itself within 1 to 2 weeks. Referral and a prescription for oral antibiotics may be necessary if no relief is seen in approximately 14 days.

Trichiasis

Trichiasis is a condition whereby the eyelashes grow inwards, causing corneal abrasion and thus affecting the eyesight. The eyelash needs to be regularly pulled out with a tweezer by a qualified health care professional, and sometimes electrolysis or cryotherapy of the hair follicles may be considered.

Watery Eyes

Watery eyes are caused by excessive tear production, a natural process that keeps the eye lubricated and clean. Allergies are a common cause of watery eyes, in addition to blepharitis and infection. The choice of treatment will be based upon the cause. Nonprescription antihistamines may be useful in preventing watery eyes related to allergy.

Xanthelasma

Xanthelasma is a frequently bilateral condition that is usually found in elderly individuals and those with hypercholesterolemia. It presents as a yellow subcutaneous plaque on the eyelids. Since it can be an indication of hypercholesterolemia, patients should be referred for a cholesterol test.

Foreign Body in the Eye

The symptoms of a foreign body include sharp pain, burning, irritation, tearing, and redness. The patient may feel something in the eye when moving the eye around while it is closed and a scratching sensation upon blinking. Bleeding may be seen in the white part of the eye and in more severe cases the vision may be affected or there may be a complete loss of vision. In less serious situations, whereby there is no corneal abrasion or loss of vision, a simple eye wash can be used to remove the foreign body.

Preservatives in Eye Care Products

Additives, such as preservatives, need to be taken into consideration when selecting an appropriate medication. Preservatives in eye drops can cause stinging and itching as well as keratitis. Furthermore, preservatives decrease the stability of the precorneal tear film and have a detergent effect on the lipid layer, worsening a dry eye. Preservatives, such as benzalkonium chloride, are taken up by contact lenses, particularly soft contact lenses. The accumulation of such preservatives eventually reaches toxic levels, causing further irritation to the eye. Patients should be advised not to wear any lenses for an hour after instilling eye drops containing preservatives.

Role of the Pharmacist

Pharmacists should demonstrate the proper use of ophthalmic drops to patients so that the medication is applied correctly. Leaflets that instruct patients on how to instill eye drops are readily available and should be used to reinforce the explanation. As a rule of thumb, any patients presenting with pain in the eye should be referred for further investigation immediately. Many symptoms, particularly dryness, watery eyes, and redness, are common to a number of ocular conditions. While pharmacists are not experts in treating eye conditions, they are in a position to give patients advice based upon the symptoms presented and explain the correct use of the medications.

With pharmacists increasingly becoming the first port of call for many patients, it is essential to have basic knowledge of common eye disorders and their management. List of possible questions the pharmacists may ask during a consultation with a patient presenting with an eye problem are listed below

List of Possible Questions

- How long have you had the problem?
- Have you had this problem before?
- What is the pattern of occurrence of this problem?

- Has it got worse or better over time?
- Is there any pain?
- Is there any discharge?
- Is your vision affected?
- Do you know what the problem could be? Is there an obvious cause?
- Have you been using a computer for prolonged periods of time?

KEY POINTS

- Pharmacists' role in treating minor ailments such as body pains & aches, dyspepsia, nausea & vomiting, gastritis, diarrhea; constipation is commonly practiced and highly appreciated.
- Pharmacist should understand the patient's symptoms and suggest suitable pharmacist only medicines to treat the clinical condition.
- Refer the patient to the doctors if situation require.

SUGGESTED READINGS

1. Annatjie Bouwer, Nausea and Vomiting – an approach for pharmacists. S Afr Pharm J 2011;78(7): 28–32.
2. Bridges S (2012). Health survey for England 2011: Chronic pain (Chapter 9). NHS Health and Social Care Information Centre.
3. Degnan R et al. The impact of face-to-face educational outreach on diarrhoea treatment in pharmacies. Health Policy and Planning, 1996, 11: 308–318.
4. Hogan R. Educating private drug sellers. Dialogue on Diarrhoea, 1994, Issue no. 55, 2–4.
5. Hogan R. Educating private drug sellers. Dialogue on Diarrhoea, 1994, Issue no. 55, 2–4. Robin Green, Prakash Jeena, Shane Kotze, et al. Management of acute fever in children: Guideline for community healthcare providers and pharmacists. South African Medical Journal. 2013. 13 (7): 984.
6. Kiran Panesar. Managing Common Eye Conditions in the Pharmacy. US Pharm.2010;35(4): 42-46.
7. Megan E Keller, David R Bright, Donald L Sullivan and Doug C Cornelius. Assessment of Community pharmacists willingness and barriers of Medication Therapy management focused on Pain management and Mental health. Innovations in Pharmacy. 2014, Vol.5: 1-5.

CHAPTER 13

HEALTH PROMOTION

LEARNING OBJECTIVES

- Understand the definition of health
- Know the techniques to promote the concept of health among the public
- Provide strategies to improve the health in children, pregnant women and geriatric patients

Health is a state of general wellbeing of an individual in all respects. It is also a level of functional and/or metabolic efficiency of a person. In 1948, World Health Organization (WHO) defined Health as ***"a state of complete physical, mental, and social well being and not merely absence of disease or infirmity"***. The La Londe report suggests that four general determinants influence the public health such as human biology, environment, lifestyle and healthcare services. Thus, health is maintained and improved not only through the advancement and application of health science but also through the efforts and intelligent lifestyle choices of the individual and the society. The Alameda County study examined the relationship between lifestyle and health. It has found that people can improve their health through exercise, enough sleep, maintaining a healthy weight, limiting the use of alcohol and avoiding smoking.

In developing countries like India, malnutrition, cigarette smoking, chewing pan masala, alcohol consumption and unhygienic living conditions are the major determinants for poor health. Illiteracy also adds to the problem. Health promotion is the strategy used to promote the concept of good health among the people.

In 2005, WHO defined health promotion as "the process of enabling people to increase control over their health and its determinants and thereby improve their health". Health promotion examines underlying economic, social, and environmental conditions, risk factors that affects and endangers the health of the individuals and communicates the health related information and skills to the individuals to lead a healthy life.

SKILLS TO IMPROVE THE HEALTH

Health of the individuals depends upon various factors like personal hygiene, personal involvement in social activities, and managing the stress in life.

Personal hygiene

Hygiene is the practice of keeping the body clean to prevent infection and illness, and avoiding contact with infectious agents. Hygiene practices include bathing, brushing and flossing teeth, washing hands especially before eating, washing fruits before they are eaten, cleaning food preparation utensils and surfaces before and after preparing meals, and many others. These practices help the individual in preventing infections and illnesses. By cleaning the body, dead skin cells are washed away with the germs, decreasing the chances of their entry in to the body.

Social activity

Personal health depends partially on the social structure of one's life. Maintenance of strong social relationships is also linked to good health, longevity, productivity. Many research studies have revealed that positive social interaction produces certain chemicals in the brain which are linked to personality and intelligence traits. Volunteering in social functions will help the individual to overcome their personal problems and lead a healthy life. Volunteering in social services will add years of life. According to a university study conducted for 7 years comparing the people who volunteered in social service with those who were not, the findings suggest that, senior citizens who have volunteered had shown a 67% reduced risk of dying.

Stress management

Modern world is posing work challenges and pressures to the individuals. Prolonged psychological stress negatively affects the health and productivity of the individual and has been cited as a factor for cognitive impairment, aging, depressive illness, and expression of psychosomatic diseases. Stress management is the application of methods to reduce stress or increase tolerance to stress. Relaxation techniques are physical methods used to relieve stress. Psychological methods include cognitive therapy, meditation, and positive thinking which work by reducing the response to stress. Improving relevant skills and abilities build confidence, which also reduces the stress reaction to situations where those skills are applicable. Learning to cope with problems better, such as improving problem solving and time management skills, may also reduce stressful reaction to problems.

HEALTH PROMOTION IN CHILDREN

From the birth to adolescence, children require adequate support from parents and elders to improve their physical and mental health. Pediatric age group ranges between 0-14 years. At different stages of the pediatric age, various health problems or health related accidents are experienced by the children. Based on their age, children are classified in to neonates, pediatrics and adolescents.

Health promotion activities in children can be divided in to:

(a) Immunization
(b) Nutrition
(c) Oral Hygiene
(d) Healthy habits

Immunization

Immunization is defined as a process by which an individual's immune system becomes fortified against an agent known as the immunogen. Immunization can be done through various techniques, most commonly by vaccination. Vaccines against microorganisms that cause diseases can prepare the body's immune system, thus helping the individual to fight or prevent an infection.

Immunization in children is very important to boost their immunity strength. Thus from their birth to till the age of the adolescence, various vaccines should be given to the children at different ages. Soon after the birth, first dose of Hepatitis B vaccine should be given and within the first month of the life, second dose should be administered. In the first 6-8 weeks of the life, first set of vaccination to diphtheria, polio, tetanus (DPT) and whooping cough should be recommended. The second set and third set of vaccinations should be administered in the 3rd and 4th month of the baby's life. The vaccination against Measles, Mumps and Rabies (MMR) are recommended at the age of 13 months of baby's life. At this age a booster dose of Hepatitis B vaccine may be recommended. At the age of 4-5 years of the child's life, once again DPT and MMR vaccines should be given.

ROLE OF COMMUNITY PHARMACISTS IN VACCINATION

Community Pharmacies are considered as the first point of contact, stock the vaccines and advice the patients suitably and refer the patients to the doctors when required. In many countries, pharmacies are the key points for disseminating messages prepared by their National authorities individually or in collaboration with National Pharmacy Associations. Pharmacists are trustworthy and authoritative sources for disease and medicines information and are trained to communicate information in such a way that empowers people to make informed and independent decisions regarding risks and benefits to their health. During the outbreak of H1N1 infection, besides the provision of information at pharmacy level, community pharmacist can play vital role in conducting health education camps in schools and other community organizations to improve the awareness of H1N1 related issues. Community pharmacists can also work as immunization facilitators and where possible under the national law, can become immunizers and take an active role in protecting vulnerable people. In some countries like Portugal, pharmacists are already involved in population vaccination for seasonal influenza; and in U.K and Ireland, pharmacists are being trained to provide H1N1 immunization. In US, pharmacists stock the vaccines and immunize the public against various infections.

Nutrition

Proper nutrition will ensure the child's normal body growth and development from the months through the teenage years. It is important to establish good eating habits from young age and children should be told about the value of avoiding high fat foods and the importance of fiber, calcium, iron and other minerals in the diet. Eating a well balanced diet from an early age has lifelong benefits.

A Child's Daily Calorie requirement

In order to maintain normal growth and good health of the baby, the child requires adequate calories, and a balanced diet that supplies a wide range of essential nutrients. Calories supply the energy needed for growth, and keep the child from feeling hungry. The number of calories a child require varies based on the child's size, growth rate and activity level. A good rule of thumb is used to calculate the calories required for children up to the age of 5 years. A base of 1,000 calories and 100 calories should be added for each year of the child's age. For example a one year-old child may require approximately 1000 + 100 calories /day and two year old child may require 1000 + 200 calories i.e. 1200 calories per day. With this simple equation, one can calculate the approximate number of calories a child requires in order to maintain normal growth. Healthy adult males need about 2500 calories a day while the average healthy woman needs about 2100 calories per day. This of course varies, depending on level of activity and the body size.

Infant Formulas

It is strongly recommended that women should breastfeed their babies. But for variety of reasons some mothers may choose formula foods for their babies. In such situations commercial iron-fortified infant formulas are the right options. Various health guidelines suggest that, babies should be fed either breast milk or formula food, or a combination of both for at least 12 months. Many "homemade" infant formulas are nutritionally inadequate, and even harmful. The commercially available infant formulas are designed to imitate the content and performance of human milk as much as scientifically possible. However, no formula foods perfectly identical neither to the breast milk, nor as perfectly designed for the baby.

Mothers should consult the doctors before using infant formula to feed the baby. Based on the baby's particular needs, the doctor may advise formulas fortified with iron and contain the recommended levels of other vitamins and minerals. Iron-fortification is important to protect the baby from developing iron deficiency anemia, a serious condition which can lead to long-term delays in mental and physical development. Additional vitamin supplements generally are not needed for formula-fed babies.

Preparing Formulas

Commercial formulas are available in a variety of forms. Ready-made types come in disposable, sterile bottles or in cans for pouring into bottles at home. Concentrated and powdered formulas are also popular, and tend to be less expensive. These need to be diluted and poured into bottles before serving. Be sure to read instructions for these types of formula foods carefully. It's very important that directions for mixing should be followed exactly. Incorrectly mixed formula can result in malnutrition if it is too much diluted. Formula which is made too much concentrated can also be dangerous as it is too difficult for a baby's system to metabolize.

For the baby's first three months, water used in formula should be sterilized by boiling it. Many people aren't aware that bottled water is not sterile. If bottled water is used to mix the baby's formula, boil it first, cool and use. No matter which type of formula is used, always check packaging for the expiry date. Discard any formula which is past due. Storage instructions should be read and followed carefully. Do not reuse formula which is leftover in the bottle after a feeding as it can easily become contaminated with bacteria. Bottles and containers used to prepare formula should be sterilized or washed in very hot soapy water to avoid contaminating the milk with germs. Never the infant formulas should be heated on the stove, or in the microwave. Excessive heat can destroy important nutrients in the milk, and can burn your baby's mouth. Formula can be served at room temperature, or warmed slightly by immersing the bottle in lukewarm water, then shaking it to distribute the heat evenly.

A Word of Caution

Mothers should never leave the baby with a propped bottle - this could cause the baby to choke. Until the baby has developed the coordination to hold the bottle by herself, mother should hold both the baby and the bottle during feeding.

Starting the Baby on Solids

At the age of 6 months, breast milk and formula foods alone are not sufficient to provide the entire range of nutrients necessary to meet the baby's needs. Solid foods contain the extra calories, iron, and other nutrients. Many doctors agree that baby should be started with solid food around 4 months, regardless of how much milk the baby is taking. Feeding the solids before 4 months isn't recommended due to inadequate growth of the intestine to digest and also difficulty in swallowing the solid foods. By the fourth month, a baby's digestive system is mature enough to handle solid food and is able to absorb nutrients supplied in solid food. However, it is recommended that babies be breastfed exclusively for the first 6 months. Parents are advised to talk to their health care professional before starting solids at a younger age. Commercial baby cereals are a good first food - they are heavily enriched with iron and important B vitamins, and are specially designed for a young baby's delicate digestive system. They are also convenient, as they're pre-cooked; the mothers need to add water, breast milk or formula, depending on the brand. If any mother chooses to use commercial cereals, be sure to read and follow mixing instructions carefully. At first, start with one teaspoon of cereal in the morning, and one at supper. Gradually increase the quantity if the baby responds well to the food. Variety of fortified cereals may be tried for new taste and sensation. Watch for any adverse reactions. Once the baby has become accustomed to cereals, at about 6 months, bland pureed vegetables such as peas or carrots may be added to her food. After a couple of weeks, variety of fruit purees may be tried. Fruit purees can be followed in later weeks by pureed chicken, meat or cottage cheese. All home-prepared foods should be pureed until your baby develops adequate mouth coordination to mash or chew. Be sure to consult the doctor about which foods are appropriate for the baby.

ROLE OF PHARMACIST IN CHILD NUTRITION

Pharmacist should stock all the necessary baby foods suiting to all age ranges of the babies. Whenever the baby foods are sold, pharmacist should educate the parents about feeding of babies, sterilization procedure, proper mixing of foods, introduction of vegetables, egg and non vegetarian soup etc., from time to time to improve the baby fitness.

Oral Health

Dental caries (tooth decay) affect 66% of five year old children and 70% of 12 year old children in general. Dental caries is identified as one of the most common reasons for hospital admissions. Periodontal (gum) disease affects majority of adults and the restoration, maintenance and prosthetic replacement of carious teeth continues throughout the life. Dental diseases are totally preventable, but are strongly influenced by lifestyle, cultural and socio-economic factors.

Oral health promotion aims at increasing the awareness about the causes and prevention of oral diseases.

ROLE OF COMMUNITY PHARMACISTS IN ORAL HYGIENE

Hidden sugars in baby foods and juices, liquid medicines, lozenges and cough sweets do enormous damage to teeth on a prolonged use. Pharmacists are ideally placed to advise the public on safe use and sugar free alternatives. Promotion of drinking cups for young children is also to be encouraged by pharmacists. Fluoride supplements, fluoride toothpaste and other topical fluorides have the ability to reduce the risk of dental caries. A pharmacist, trained in oral health, can advise the public on the most appropriate choices and use of fluoride preparations.

Pharmacists should give an advice on denture hygiene and also encourage annual attendance at the dentist for oral cancer screening. Mouth ulcers and other soft tissue lesions presented to the pharmacist for advice are usually benign. A pharmacist's advice and early referral to a dentist can reduce the risk of malignancy progressing undetected. Recurrent ulcers can also be a marker for other health problems. The pharmacist should give proper advice directly to the patient and encourage them for a dentist referral in case of frequent or persistent oral health problems. Pharmacists' analgesic service is much appreciated during emergencies and out of hour dental practice. Pharmacists' involvement in the dental camps such as "National Smile Week" certainly recognizes the pharmacist as health care provider.

Healthy Habits in Children

Early childhood is an ideal time to motivate the children to establish healthy habits or behaviors that will promote healthy lifestyles. It is essential for all of us to teach kids to stay healthy. In order to develop healthy habits two things must be remembered. First learning becomes more meaningful when the experience is woven into the children's daily experiences. Second, learning experiences must be repeated often enough until the lessons become a natural and integral part of their lives. Following are the good habits the children need to be trained.

Good Hand Washing

Children during their school hours often touch the tables, desks or other objects which are dirty and contaminated. Children often tend to eat foods without proper hand wash and that may make them sick due to infections. Good hand washing using soap, water and friction will remove the dirt and kill all germs and make the hands clean and sterilized. Everyone should wash hands before and after eating, or using the bathroom, or handling nappies, or blowing into a handkerchief or tissue, or cleaning, or doing art projects, or playing with toys. Proper hand washing can significantly reduce transmission of infections.

Getting Enough Sleep

Another healthy habit that kids must develop is to get enough sleep. Studies show lack of sufficient sleep can contribute to poor attention, hyperactivity, and adamant among the children. Most children's sleep requirements fall within a predictable range of hours based on their age. However, there is no magical number of sleeping hours required as each child would have his own distinct sleep needs.

Eating Healthy Food

Good nutrition is a wonderful foundation for wellness. Everyone needs to eat variety of foods to maintain their health. Vegetables, fruits, milk, cheese, fish, chicken, meat, nuts, rice and grains are the good foods for children. A balanced diet is one that includes all the food groups. Not many of us eat a balanced diet on a regular basis. More so are children who frequently skip the meals. Toddlers and preschoolers are often picky about the food they eat. Taking a multi vitamin/multi mineral supplement will ensure that they are well-nourished and are getting the nutrients they need for normal growth and development.

Exercise

Most kids are active and if they are encouraged to stay healthy by developing their love for exercise and activities that make them move. Physical activity should be increased by reducing sedentary time (e.g., watching television, playing computer video games or talking on the phone.) All children in the age of two years or old should participate in at least 30 minutes of enjoyable, moderate-intensity activities every day and be sure they drink plenty of water.

Health Promotion and Care for Pregnant Women and Breast Feeding Mothers

Pregnancy is often considered as a second birth to the pregnant lady. Proper medical care during pregnancy is vital for both mother and fetus health. Historically, prenatal care has been one of the most significant factors in saving mother's life and decreasing fetal mortality. Although variety of over-the-counter tests can confirm the pregnancy, however a gynecologist can detect the pregnancy as early as eight to nine days after fertilization. During the first visit, the doctor may evaluate the health of the woman and fetus. Her blood pressure, height, and weight will be measured, and blood & urine samples will be tested for susceptibility to infection, maternal blood type, and the presence of certain other diseases. The gynecologist may perform a pelvic examination to measure the size of the woman's womb. The age of the fetus in "weeks of gestation completed" will be estimated from the woman's last menstrual period. This help the consultant to determine the delivery date and provide ideal prenatal care.

The gynecologist may further advise the woman on diet, relaxation and sleep, exercise, and the dangers of smoking, drinking, and using the OTC drugs. Nutritional counseling is an important part of prenatal care as eating well during pregnancy is essential to the health of the growing fetus. The first visit ends with an individualized plan for continued care. This may range from routine visits to specialized or intensive care if necessary. It is best for both woman and fetus when, even before pregnancy, a woman takes care of her body by eating well, exercising, and avoiding harmful substances. Initiating prenatal care as early as possible promotes maternal and fetal health. The fetus health can only be maximized by improving the mother's health. The ultimate goal of this care is to enable a mother to safely deliver a healthy baby.

After the delivery, breast feeding benefits both mother and the baby. "Clostrum" the first milk of the mother posses unique antibodies which gives the protection to the baby from various infections. Many studies have revealed that, breast feeding increases the attachment of baby with the mother and also the self esteem to the mother and also prevent the possibilities of breast cancer.

ROLE OF THE PHARMACIST IN COUNSELING THE PREGNANT WOMEN

Pharmacists may help the pregnant women by dispensing the quality medicines and educating the women about safe use of medicines. The pharmacist should advise the woman on diet, relaxation, sleep, exercise, dangers of smoking, drinking, and using OTC and other drugs. Nutritional counseling is an important part of prenatal care as eating balanced diet during pregnancy will improve the health of the growing fetus. The ultimate goal of this care is to enable a mother to safely deliver a healthy baby. After the delivery, the mothers should be advised about the importance of breast milk and also suitable advice may be given regarding the formula feeds. Certain medications are excreted in the breast milk. Thus the nursing mothers suitably advised regarding the breast feeding while on these medications.

Health Promotion in Geriatrics

India is witnessing a demographic transition, leading to a rapid increase in the number of elderly people. Average life expectancy has increased and is around 64 years and the longevity is expected to enhance further. During 2001, India was the second largest in having more number of elderly (60+) in the world and likely to constitute 17.5% of the total elderly of the world by 2050. The increasing longevity in India is now posing new challenges for ensuring the well-being of the huge number of the elderly. One of the main factors that determine the well-being at old age is the chronic non communicable disease (NCD). However, empirical evidences suggest that the disability and adverse consequences of NCD can be prevented or postponed by health and fitness promotion throughout the life. Thereby, it will be possible to maximize the period of healthy life expectancy. NCDs usually occur later in life, but the risk of most NCDs begins at childhood or adolescence, or even in *uterus* through maternal health during pregnancy. Hence, chronic diseases in the adult or in the elderly reflect cumulative life-time exposures to risk factors. Thus a strategy to counter preventable NCD risk factors through life-course approach remains as one of the major targets to improve quality of life at old age.

Physical inactivity, unhealthy diet (diet with high calorie, sugar, saturated fats, salt, less intake of fruit and vegetables), tobacco use, and alcohol intake are components of lifestyle that contribute to a large fraction of NCDs in the population. Chronic NCDs by themselves are a series of overlapping and complicated disease entities; and they share many common risk factors. Tobacco use is one of the most important risk factors of four important NCDs (cancer, heart diseases, stroke, Chronic Obstructive Pulmonary Disease (COPD)). Physical inactivity and unhealthy diets are risk factors of a group of inter-related NCDs like diabetes, coronary heart disease (CHD) and stroke. Hence, all of them can be postponed, cost effectively by an integrated approach.

However, available data in India indicate that the gain in life expectancy is going to be accompanied by increased years of poor health due to chronic diseases, resulting in 'expansion of morbidity' rather than 'compression'. India is experiencing a rapid health transition with NCD emerging as the number one disease burden replacing 'pre-transitional' diseases. India is known as the 'diabetes capital of the world' and also bear the burden of quarter of the world's CHD. Further, the amplifying role of diabetes for other serious NCDs is also an important concern for the country. Many cancers linked to preventable hazardous lifestyle are reported to be high in India. Early age of occurrence of diabetes and CHD has been recorded among Indians compared to the developed countries; hence survivors of these diseases face associated disability at a much earlier age.

Although genetic component plays an important role in early occurrence of NCDs, modifiable lifestyle factors are also considered as the primary driving force of NCDs in India. Rapid urbanization, modernization and its accompanying adverse lifestyle changes e.g., tobacco/alcohol use, unhealthy food habits, sedentary lifestyle along with population ageing are influencing the increased burden of NCDs. Thus, there is an urgent need to intensify NCD prevention efforts in India. World Health Organization also recommended life course approach in dealing with increasing NCDs and emphasized positive interventions in earlier life.

ROLE OF PHARMACIST IN GERIATRIC CARE

Ageing is a natural phenomenon. As the age advances, both physical and psychological health related problems increases in the elderly individuals. Decreased functioning of the internal organs, physical debility, various other diseases such as hypertension, diabetes, asthma, urological problems and psychological stress makes individuals more badly. In such situations, if pharmacists' counsels the senior citizens about the diseases and medications will improve their understanding about the medication adherence behavior and disease management. Monitoring their health through screening services such as checking blood pressure and blood sugar will give them confidence about their therapy. A positive motivation about good hygiene improves healthy behavior. Often forming senior citizen clubs, conducting group counseling and peer sharing of the strategies to manage the diseases will have positive effect in controlling many chronic disorders. Home medication review program and discussing with the patient's doctor about the drug related problems and the strategies to minimize them will further strengthen the elderly health care.

KEY POINTS

- Health promotion is a strategic approach to improve the public health by influencing the health determinants.
- Pharmacists have a definite role in health promotion through public education regarding immunization, formula feeds, non-communicable diseases, and safe use of medicines.

SUGGESTED READINGS

1. Andy Stergachis, Roger D. Lander, Lauren E. Webb. Promoting pharmacist role in public health. J Am Pharm Assoc (2003) 2006; 46: 311-319.
2. Community Pharmacists and Health Promotion. A study on consultations between pharmacists and clients. Health Promotion international. Vol.7 (4): 249-255.
3. Public Health- A Practical Guide for community pharmacists. Accessed through internet: http://psnc.org.uk/wp-content/uploads/2013/07/public_health_book_all.pdf
4. Role of pharmacists in screening and prevention. The Translator. Canandian Pharmacists Association. 2012.

CHAPTER **14**

BALANCE DIET, TREATMENT AND PREVENTION OF DEFICIENCY DISORDERS

LEARNING OBJECTIVES

- Know the definition and composition of balanced diet
- Understand the various nutritional deficiency disorders.
- Appreciate the role of pharmacist in diet counseling

INTRODUCTION

Nutrition is the intake of food in relation to the body's dietary requirements. Good nutrition is an adequate, well balanced diet combined with regular physical activity. Good nutrition is the cornerstone for good health. Poor nutrition may affect the body's immunity, increases susceptibility to diseases, impair the physical and mental growth and reduce an individual's productivity. A well balanced diet maintains the general health of the individuals. A "Balanced Diet" is a mixture of macro and micro nutrients that provide adequate energy to the individual to carry out the day today activities. As per Thesaurus, the balanced diet is defined as the diet that contains adequate amounts of all the necessary nutrients required for healthy growth and activity.

Composition of Balanced Diet

A Balanced diet is defined as the diet that contains the required amount of calories, vitamins and minerals that are essential to keep a person healthy. A balanced diet is a mix of Carbohydrates (50%), Fats (32%), Proteins (12%), Minerals and Vitamins (3%) and sufficient water.

Objectives of the Balanced Diet

Following are the objectives of the balanced diet:

(a) The diet should keep the person healthy.

(b) It should offer the individuals sufficient energy to do their normal routine work.

World Health Organisation (WHO) gave the following five recommendations to individuals regarding the balanced diet:

1. Individuals are advised to burn as much energy as a person can, and try to eat as much to maintain a healthy weight.
2. Increase the consumption of food producing plants, particularly fruits and vegetables, legumes, whole grains and nuts.
3. Limit the intake of fat and oil, and avoid saturated fats which are those that become solid at room temperature such as coconut oil and all animal products including meat, dairy products and eggs. Prefer unsaturated fats which remain liquid at room temperature instead, and which are found in almost all the plant based oils and foods. Eliminate trans- fatty acids.
4. Limit the intake of granulated sugar.
5. Limit salt/sodium consumption from all sources and ensure that salt is iodized

Other Suggested Recommendations

Eat fish or animal meat or soya beans sufficient to have cellular replenishment and transport proteins. All essential amino acids are present only in animals. However people skip meat products from their diets may still easily obtain all the essential amino acid in their diets by consuming adequate amounts of plant products and grain products, which combine to provide complete proteins to the diet. Fruits such as avocado and pumpkin seeds also have almost all of the essential amino acids.

- Take essential micronutrients such as vitamins and certain minerals through suitable foods that can offer them.

Nutrition Deficiency Disorders

Nutritional deficiency disorders include: protein-energy malnutrition disorders, vitamin deficiency, iodine deficiency and iron deficiency anemia.

Proteins/fats/carbohydrates

Protein-energy malnutrition disorder

- Kwashiorkor
- Marasmus
- Mental retardation

Dietary vitamins and minerals

Calcium deficiency disorder

- Osteoporosis
- Rickets
- Tetany

Iodine deficiency disorder

- Goiter

Iron Deficiency Disorder

Iron deficiency anemia

- Thiamine (Vitamin B_1)
    - Beriberi
- Niacin (Vitamin B_3)
    - Pellagra
- Vitamin C
    - Scurvy
- Vitamin D
    - Osteoporosis
    - Rickets

Protein Deficiency Disorders

1. **Kwashiorkar: "Kwashiorkar"** was first identified by a Jamaican pediatrician Dr. Cicely Williams in young children as an acute form of protein-energy malnutrition characterized by edema, irritability, anorexia, ulcerating dermatoses and an enlarged liver with fatty infiltrates. This situation develops in young children when the mother replaces the breast milk which is rich in proteins and vital amino acids with diet rich in carbohydrates. As a result of insufficient protein consumption, but with sufficient calorie intake, kwashiorkor develops. Kwashiorkor cases are often seen in areas of poor food supply.

   Signs and symptoms: The signs and symptoms of Kwashiorkar are

    1. Typical ulcerating dermatosis
    2. Pedal edema (swelling of the feet)
    3. Distended abdomen
    4. An enlarged liver with fatty infiltrates,
    5. Thinning hair
    6. Loss of teeth,
    7. Skin depigmentation and dermatitis.
    8. Irritability
    9. Anorexia.

Victims of Kwashiorkor fail to produce antibodies following vaccination against diseases, including diphtheria and typhoid. Generally, the disease can be treated by adding protein to the diet; however, it can have a long-term impact on a child's physical and mental development, and in severe cases this may lead to death.

Management: The children affected with Kwashiorkar should be fed with dietary protein gradually

2. **Marasmus:** The word **"Marasmus"** comes from the Greek *marasmos* ("decay") and is defined as the gradual wasting away of the body due to severe malnutrition or inadequate absorption of food. Marasmus is a form of severe protein deficiency and is one of the forms of protein-energy malfunction (PEM).

   The children with marasmus look emaciated and body weight may be reduced to less than 80% of the average weight that corresponds to the height. Marasmus is often seen prior to one year of age, whereas kwashiorkor is seen after 18 months of age. Marasmus can be distinguished from kwashiorkor through symptoms of protein wasting with the presence of edema. The prognosis is better than the kwashiorkor disease.

   Signs and symptoms: The malnutrition associated with marasmus leads to extensive tissue and muscle wasting, as well as variable edema. Other common signs and symptoms include

   1. Dry skin,
   2. Loose skin folds hanging over the buttocks (glutei) and arm pit (axillae) etc.
   3. Drastic loss of adipose tissue from normal areas of fat deposits like buttocks and thighs.
   4. Fretful, Irritable, and voraciously hungry.

   Causes: Marasmus is caused by a severe deficiency of nearly all nutrients, especially protein and carbohydrates.

   Treatment: It is necessary to treat not only the symptoms but also the complications of the disorder, including infections, dehydration, and circulation disorders, which are frequently lethal and lead to high mortality if ignored.

3. *Cachexia (wasting syndrome):* Cachexia is defined as a state of weight loss, muscle atrophy, fatigue, weakness, and significant loss of appetite due to some pathological involvement. Cachexia physically weakens the patients to a state of immobility starting from loss of appetite, asthenia, and anemia. The patients with Cachexia will respond poorly to standard treatment. Cachexia is seen in patients with cancer, AIDS, chronic obstructive lung disease, multiple sclerosis, congestive heart failure, tuberculosis, familial amyloid polyneuropathy, mercury poisoning (acrodynia) and hormonal deficiency. Cachexia is considered as a positive risk factor for death.

   Mechanism: The exact mechanism for Cachexia in various disorders is poorly understood, however a probable role of inflammatory cytokines, such as TNF alpha, interferon gamma and interleukin 6, as well as the tumor-secreted proteolysis-inducing factors is considered in causing Cachexia.

   Treatment: Currently, no FDA-approved drugs are available to treat Cachexia. Cachexia may be treated by steroids, such as corticosteroids, or drugs that mimic progesterone, which increase appetite, may reverse weight loss, but have no evidence of reversing muscle loss.

OMEGA-3 FATTY ACIDS

A systematic review of n-3 fatty acids and Cachexia concluded an evidence of oral n-3 fatty acid supplements benefiting cancer patients, improving appetite, weight and quality of life. A 2009 trial found a supplement of eicosapentaenoic acid helped cancer patients to retain the muscle mass.

Vitamin Deficiency Disorders

Vitamins are organic components in food that are needed in very small amounts for growth and maintaining of good health. First time the term "Vitamin" was coined in 1912 by the polish bio chemist Kazimierz Funk.

All vitamins are classified in to 1) Fat soluble vitamins e.g., A, D, E and K. 2) Water soluble vitamins e.g., B- Complex and Vitamin C.

Functions of Vitamins

Vitamins have diverse biochemical functions such as

1. Hormone-in regulating mineral metabolism e.g., vitamin D
2. Regulator of cell and tissue growth and differentiation (e.g., some forms of vitamin A)
3. Antioxidants (e.g., vitamin E and sometimes vitamin C)
4. Precursors for enzyme cofactors that help enzymes in their work as catalysts in metabolism e.g., Vitamin B Complex.

VITAMIN DEFICIENCY DISORDERS

Vitamin A Deficiency Disorder

Vitamin A deficiency is lack of vitamin A in the human body. Night blindness is the first sign of vitamin A deficiency. Vitamin A play a major role in phototransduction and its deficiency may result in xerophthalmia, keratomalacia, and complete blindness. Every year approximately 2-5 lakh children from developing countries are suffering from Vitamin A deficiency and half of them die within a year due to blindness. Prevalence of night blindness due to vitamin A deficiency is also high among pregnant women in many developing countries. Studies have also shown that maternal mortality and other poor outcomes in pregnancy and lactation may occur due to Vitamin A deficiency.

Functions of Vitamin A

Vitamin A plays several roles in the body for

- Vision
- Gene transcription
- Immune function
- Embryonic development and reproduction

- Bone metabolism
- Haematopoiesis
- Skin and cellular health
- Antioxidant activity

Signs and Symptoms

Vitamin A deficiency may cause

- Night blindness,
- Xerophthalmia,
- Keratomalacia
- Complete blindness
- Impaired immune function
- Birth defects

Causes Vitamin A Deficiency

- Lactating mother with vitamin A deficiency contains little vitamin A, which provides a breast-fed child with too little vitamin A.
- Iron deficiency can affect vitamin A uptake.
- Excess alcohol consumption can deplete vitamin A

Management

Deficiency of Vitamin A can be achieved by eating vitamin A rich foods and external supplementation of Vitamin A preparations.

Vitamin A Dupplementation

The average daily requirement of Vitamin A for children is 300-600 µg, for adults is 700 µg to 900 µg (3000 IU) and for lactating mothers the daily requirement is 1500-1800 µg (5000 IU to 6000 IU).

Foods Rich in Vitamin A

Vitamin A is found naturally in many foods:

- Liver (beef, pork, chicken, turkey, fish) (6500 µg), including cod liver oil
- Dandelion greens (5588 IU)
- Carrot (835 µg)
- Broccoli leaf (800 µg)
- Sweet Potato (709 µg)
- Butter (684 µg)
- Spinach (469 µg)

- Pumpkin (400 µg)
- Cheddar cheese (265 µg)
- Egg (140 µg)
- Apricot (96 µg)
- Papaya (55 µg)
- Mango (38 µg)
- Pea (38 µg)
- Milk (28 µg)

Vitamin D Deficiency Disorder

Vitamin D is a group of fat-soluble secosteroids and is also called as sunshine vitamin. In humans when sun exposure is adequate, vitamin D is synthesized from the body cholesterol. Vitamin D can be ingested as Cholecalciferol (vitamin D_3) or Ergocalciferol (vitamin D_2). In the liver, Vitamin D is converted in to calcidiol and is further converted in to calcitriol in the kidneys which is biologically active form of Vitamin D. Calcitriol circulates in the blood as a hormone regulating the concentration of calcium and phosphate in blood and promote the healthy growth and remodeling of bone. Calcidiol is also converted to Calcitriol outside of the kidneys for other purposes, such as the proliferation, differentiation and apoptosis of cells. Calcitriol also affects neuromuscular function and inflammation.

Functions of Vitamin D

The important functions of vitamin D are:

1. Maintain the normal calcium and phosphorus levels in the body to build strong bones, teeth and nails.
2. Supporting the cell functions and other neuromuscular functions in the body.
3. Controls the supply of calcium between the bones and the blood and supports bone mineralization (hardening of bones) and bone remodeling by osteoblasts and osteoclasts.
4. Preventing of rickets in children, and osteoporosis or osteomalacia in adults.
5. Vitamin D as a powerful antioxidant and anti-carcinogen, it helps in combating depression, prostate cancer, breast cancer, high blood pressure, cardiovascular diseases, phagocytosis activity and boosts anti-tumor activity.
6. Vitamin D also helps treating conditions like diabetes and obesity, and prevents the onset of multiple sclerosis.
7. Vitamin D helps in maintaining a healthy immune system in the body.

Sources of Vitamin D

The main source of vitamin D is exposure of an individual is to the sun's UVB rays. Apart from this, Vitamin D is found in various types of fish such as herring, mackerel, salmon, and sardines. It is also available in other food sources such as egg yolks, orange juice, cereals, green leafy vegetables, fish liver oils, yogurt, cheese, etc. Fortified foods are other common sources of vitamin D. In fact, one cup of vitamin D fortified milk provides one-half of the recommended vitamin D for people between the ages of 19 and 50 years.

Vitamin D Deficiency Disorders

A diet deficient in vitamin D causes osteomalacia (softening of the bones) in elders and rickets in children. Avoiding the exposure to sun may result in low blood Calcidiol (25-hydroxy-vitamin D) and that may cause Vitamin D deficiency disorder.

Management

Dietary supplementation of Vitamin D_2 (Mushrooms) and Vitamin D_3 (Fish liver oils, Egg and Beef liver.

Vitamin E Deficiency Disorder

Vitamin E is a group of eight fat-soluble compounds that include both tocopherols and tocotrienols. Among the tocopherols, α-Tocopherol is biologically active form of vitamin E. tocotrienols is much less studied. Some in vivo studies have observed that tocotrienols have specialized roles in protecting neurons from damage and cholesterol reduction by inhibiting the activity of HMG-CoA reductase, delta-tocotrienol blocks processing of sterol regulatory element-binding proteins (SREBPs). Oral consumption of tocotrienols is also thought to protect against stroke-associated brain damage

Dietary Sources

Vitamin E is found most abundantly in wheat germ oil, sunflower oil, safflower oil, nuts and nut oils, like almonds and hazelnuts, palm oil. It is also found in high-value green, leafy vegetables like spinach, turnip, broccoli, avocados, asparagus, kiwifruit (green), pumpkin, sweet potato, mangoes, tomatoes, rockfish, and papaya. It is an antioxidant that stops the production of reactive oxygen species formed when fat undergoes oxidation.

Functions

Vitamin E has following functions:

1. Prevents the oxidative damage of the cell membranes
2. Prevents unnecessary growth of the smooth muscle.
3. Responsible for the repair of wounds.
4. Vitamin E plays a role in neurological functions
5. It inhibits platelet aggregation.
6. Vitamin E also protects lipids and prevents the oxidation of polyunsaturated fatty acids (PUFAs.)

Deficiency Disorders of Vitamin E

Dietary deficiency of Vitamin E causes

- Spinocerebellar ataxia
- Myopathies
- Peripheral neuropathy
- Ataxia
- Skeletal myopathy
- Retinopathy
- Impairment of the immune response
- Erythrocyte hemolysis
- Male infertility.

Treatment

Individuals who cannot absorb fat may require a vitamin E supplement because some dietary fat is needed for the absorption of vitamin E from the gastrointestinal tract. Anyone diagnosed with cystic fibrosis, individuals who have had part or all of their stomach removed, and individuals with malabsorptive problems such as Crohn's disease, liver disease or pancreatic insufficiency may not absorb fat and may require supplemental vitamin E.

Dose of Vitamin E

The recommended dietary allowance (RDA) for vitamin E is quite low, 15 to 20 International Units (IU) per day. The most commonly recommended dosage of supplemental vitamin E for adults is approximately 300 to 800 IU per day.

Vitamin K Deficiency Disorder

Vitamin K is an essential, lipid-soluble vitamin that plays a key role in the production of coagulation proteins. Vitamin K is a mixture of three types. They are K-1 (also known as phylloquinone or phytonadione), which is derived from plants; K-2 (menaquinone), which is produced by the intestinal flora; and K-3 (menadione), which is a synthetic, water-soluble form commonly used for treatment. Estimated daily requirement of Vitamin K is 100-200 mcg/day. About 80-85% of Vitamin K is absorbed mainly in the terminal ileum into the lymphatic system; therefore, bile salts and normal fat absorption, as well as normal-functioning villi of the ileum, are necessary for the effective uptake of Vitamin K.

Symptoms of Vitamin K Deficiency

Symptoms Vitamin K deficiency include ecchymosis, petechiae, hematomas, oozing of blood at surgical or puncture sites, stomach pains; risk of massive uncontrolled bleeding; cartilage calcification; and severe malformation of developing bone or deposition of insoluble calcium salts in the walls of arteries. In infants, it can cause some birth defects such as underdeveloped face, nose, bones, and fingers.

Dietary Sources of Vitamin K

Vitamin K is found in green, leafy vegetables and in oils, such as soyabean, cottonseed, canola, and olive oils. It can also be synthesized from colonic bacteria. Diet is the main source of Vitamin K.

Deficiency Disorders of Vitamin B complex

Vitamin B complex is a group of water-soluble vitamins, easily dispersed throughout the body. Most of the B vitamins must be replenished regularly, since any excess is excreted in the urine. This can result in the production of bright green-yellow color urine. The B complex vitamin was once thought to be a single vitamin, referred to as vitamin B. However the research findings have suggested that they are chemically distinct and often coexist in the same foods. B vitamin supplements are referred as B complex named specifically by different names for each vitamin (e.g., B1, B2, B3 etc.). Following are the vitamin B Complex.

- Vitamin B1 (thiamine)
- Vitamin B2 (riboflavin)
- Vitamin B3 (niacin)
- Vitamin B5 (pantothenic acid)
- Vitamin B6 (pyridoxine)
- Vitamin B7 (biotin)
- Vitamin B9 (folic acid)
- Vitamin B12 (Cyanocobalamin)

Functions of Vitamin B Complex

The Vitamin B Complex is essential to

- Support and increase the rate of metabolism
- Maintain healthy skin, hair and muscle tone
- Enhance immune and nervous system functions
- Promote cell growth and division, including that of the red blood cells that help prevent anemia
- Reduce the risk of pancreatic cancer
- Reduce the symptoms of attention deficit hyperactivity disorder.

Deficiency Disorder of B Complex Vitamins

Several diseases may result due to inadequate intake of B vitamin supplements. Deficiencies of B - Complex vitamins result in symptoms that are not part of a named deficiency disease.

Dietary Sources of Vitamin B Complex

B-Complex vitamins are found in whole unprocessed foods. Processed carbohydrates such as sugar and white flour tend to have lower B vitamin than their unprocessed counterparts. For this reason, thiamine, riboflavin, niacin, and folic acid is added to white flour after processing. B vitamins are richly present in tuna and turkey meat and in fish liver. Good sources for B vitamins include whole grains, potatoes, bananas, lentils, chilli peppers, tempeh, beans, nutritional yeast, brewer's yeast, and molasses.

Vitamin	Name	Deficiency effects
Vitamin B1	Thiamine	**Beriberi**. Symptoms include weight loss, emotional disturbances, Wernicke's encephalopathy (impaired sensory perception), weakness and pain in the limbs, irregular heartbeat, and edema. Heart failure and death may occur in advanced cases. Chronic thiamine deficiency can also cause Korsakoff's syndrome, an irreversible psychosis characterized by amnesia and confabulation.
Vitamin B2	Riboflavin	**Ariboflavinosis**. Symptoms include cheilosis (cracks in the lips), high sensitivity to sunlight, angular cheilitis, glossitis (inflammation of the tongue), seborrheic dermatitis or pseudo-syphilis (particularly affecting the scrotum or labia majora and the mouth), pharyngitis (sore throat), hyperemia, and edema of the pharyngeal and oral mucosa.
Vitamin B3	Niacin	**Pellagra**. Symptoms include aggression, dermatitis, insomnia, weakness, mental confusion, and diarrhea. In advanced cases, pellagra may lead to dementia and death
Vitamin B5	Pantothenic acid	Deficiency can result in acne and paresthesia
Vitamin B6	Pyridoxine	Deficiency may lead to microcytic anemia, depression, dermatitis, high blood pressure (hypertension), water retention, and elevated levels of homocysteine.
Vitamin B7	Biotin	Deficiency does not typically cause symptoms in adults but may lead to impaired growth and neurological disorders in infants.
Vitamin B9	Folic acid	Deficiency results in a macrocytic anemia, and elevated levels of homocysteine.
Vitamin B12	Cobalamin	Deficiency results in a macrocytic anemia, elevated homocysteine, peripheral neuropathy, memory loss and other cognitive deficits. It can also cause symptoms of mania and psychosis. In rare extreme cases, paralysis can result.

Daily requirement of Vitamin B Complex

On individual basis, Vitamin B complex is required in different doses. However elderly people and athletes may require additional B_{12} and other Vitamin B supplementation. Both type 1 and type 2 diabetics may require thiamine based supplementation. This is may be due to high prevalence of low plasma thiamine concentration and increased thiamine clearance associated with diabetes. Also, Vitamin B_9 (folic acid) deficiency in early embryo development has been linked to neural tube defects. Thus, women planning to become pregnant are usually encouraged to increase daily dietary folic acid intake and/or take a supplement.

KEY POINTS

1. Vitamins are micronutrients essential for many metabolic reactions in the body and tissue growth.
2. Vitamin A, D, E and K are fat soluble and B Complex is water soluble vitamins.
3. Intake of right sources of foods relieves many vitamin deficiency disorders.

SUGGESTED READINGS

1. Dwyer JT. Nutrition guidelines and education of the public. J Nutr 131(11S): S3074–S3077, 2001.
2. Peckenpaugh NJ. Guides for good food choices in a family meal environment. In: Peckenpaugh NJ. Nutrition essentials and diet therapy, 9th ed. St. Louis: WB Saunders, 20033–20035.
3. Sardesai VM. Obesity and eating disorders. In: Sardesai VM. Introduction to clinical nutrition, 2nd ed. New York: Marcel Dekker, Inc., 2003: 317–337.

CHAPTER 15

FAMILY PLANNING-ROLE OF PHARMACIST

LEARNING OBJECTIVES

- Know the objectives of family planning.
- Understand various methods of family planning.
- Appreciate the role of pharmacist in family planning.

Family planning is often used as a synonym for birth control and usually applied to the circumstance of couples who wish to space between the children they want to have. Family planning is a technique that delays the pregnancy rather than preventing the pregnancy entirely. World Health Organization (WHO) defines 'family planning' as a way of living and thinking that is adopted voluntarily upon the basis of knowledge, attitudes and responsible decisions of individuals and couples in order to promote the health and welfare of the family group and thus contributes effectively to the social development of a country. WHO has appreciated the role of pharmacists in educating the patients' about advantages of family planning and useful techniques the couple can adopt suiting to their family conditions.

OBJECTIVES OF FAMILY PLANNING

Following are the objectives of family planning.

- To avoid unwanted births
- To bring about wanted births
- To regulate intervals between the pregnancies
- To determine the number of children in the family
- To control pregnancies in relation to the age of the parent
- To prevent the frequent pregnancies induced stress on the physical and psychological health of the mother.

CONTRACEPTIVE METHODS

Dated back to the history, individuals adopted various techniques to prevent the pregnancy. Various oldest forms of birth control included coitus interruptus, and the ingestion of herbs that were believed to be abortifacients. The earliest records of birth control use were found in Egypt about the use of a contraceptive pessary. Various methods are practiced currently to prevent unwanted pregnancies temporally or permanently. However a contraceptive method should be safe, effective, acceptable, and easy to use and should be economical to the user.

CLASSIFICATION OF CONTRACEPTIVE METHODS

A. Temporary methods (spacing methods)

1. Barrier methods
    - Physical methods
    - Chemical methods
    - Combined methods
2. Intra uterine devices (IUD)
3. Hormonal contraceptives
4. Post conceptual methods
5. Miscellaneous

B. Permanent methods

Male sterilization (vasectomy)

Female sterilization (Tubectomy)

Temporary Methods

1. **Barrier methods:** Barrier methods are available for both sexes. The mechanism of action is that they prevent the union of ovum with sperm either mechanically or chemically.

Physical methods: These include condom, diaphragm, and vaginal sponge.

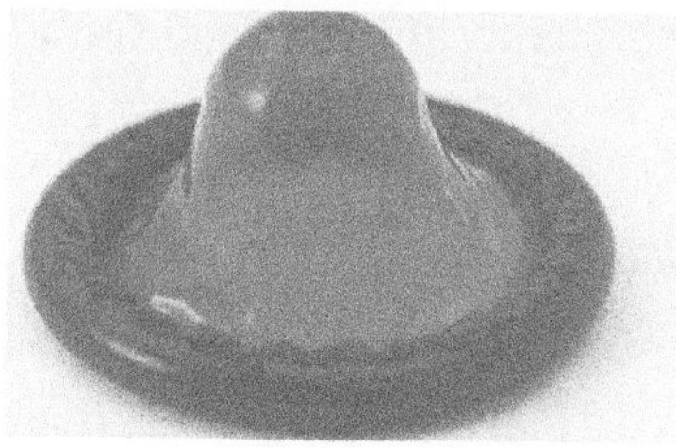

Condom: It is a male contraceptive made from latex. Some condoms are coated with a dry lubricant or with spermicide. Different sizes, shapes, colors and textures may be available. It fits over a man's erect penis.

Precautions

- Must be free from tears and leaks
- Must be discarded after single use

Advantages:

- Inexpensive
- Safe

- Easy to use and reliable
- Gives protection against STD and AIDS
- No side effects
- Light, compact and easily disposable
- It is safe and has no hormonal side effects.
- Can be used by men of all ages.

Disadvantages: Latex used to manufacture condoms or the lubricants used in the condoms may cause itching in few individuals who are allergic to latex or the lubricants.

- Incorrect use of the condom may slip off or tear during the coitus
- Some men have expressed that condom interferes with their sexual pleasure.

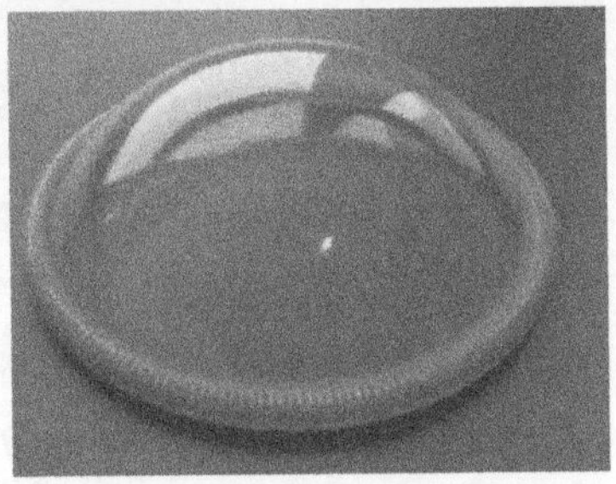

Diaphragm

It is a vaginal barrier used by women made of a synthetic rubber or plastic material. It has a flexible ring made of spring. It is inserted in to the vagina before coitus.

Precautions

- The diaphragm must remain in place for not less than six hours after the intercourse

Advantages

- Total absence of risks and medical contraindications

Disadvantages

- Initially the physician or a trained person's support is required to demonstrate the method of insertion
- Privacy is required for the insertion
- If it is left in the vagina for a longer period, it may produce a toxic shock syndrome

Vaginal Sponge

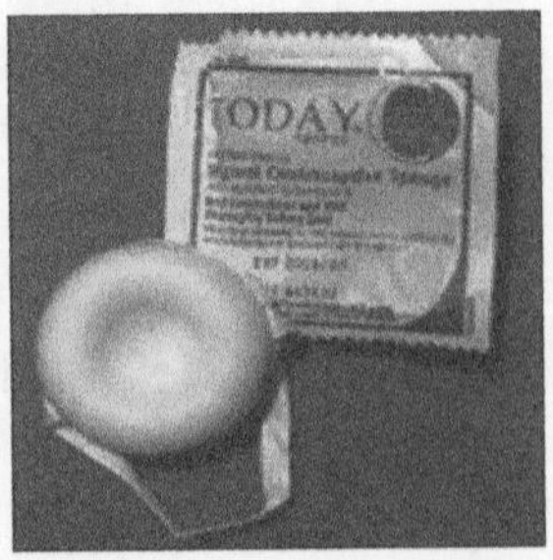

It is a small polyurethane sponge saturated with spermicidal, monoxynol-9. It is put in vagina just before coitus.

Disadvantages: Less effective than diaphragm

Chemical Methods

They make use of chemical spermicidal agents. They are used in the form of

- Foams

- Creams, pastes, jellies
- Suppositories
- Soluble film

Mechanism: The preparations contain surface active agents, which attach to the spermatozoa and inhibit the oxygen uptake thereby killing the sperms.

Advantages: Safe, and every needy woman can use because they are all woman controlled methods.

- Helps in preventing some of the sexually transmitted diseases.

Disadvantages

- High failure rate
- Mild irritation, burning and uneasiness
- Must be used immediately before coitus

Physical and chemical methods alone cannot be useful, can be used in combination called combined method to reduce the failure rate.

2. **Intra-Uterine Devices (IUD):** An intrauterine device (IUD) usually is a small, flexible plastic frame.

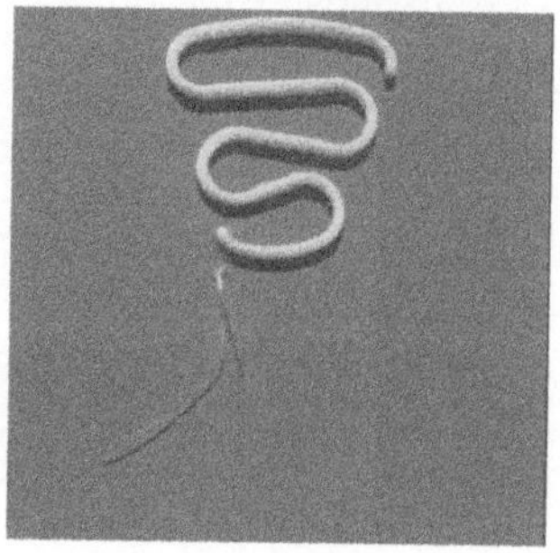

Types of IUD

First generation IUD's: They are made of polythene and they are inert and non- medicated. They appear in various sizes and shapes like loops, spirals, coils and rings. Lippes loop is commonly used one which is available in an S shaped device.

Advantages

- Simple and easy insertion
- Economical
- Reversible method
- Does not interfere with sexual pleasure

Disadvantages

- Needs a trained person for insertion
- Needs adequate follow up
- Should be replaced periodically
- Rarely it can produce cancer of uterus and fibroid

Second generation IUD

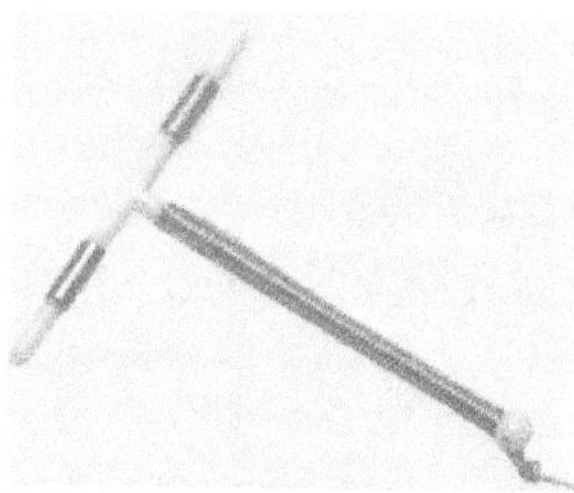

These are copper containing devices. Older devices are copper-7 and copper –T-200, newer ones are Nova-T and multi loaded devices.

Advantages

- Low expulsion rate
- Lower evidence of side effects like pain and bleeding
- Easier to fit even in nulliparous women
- Increased contraceptive effect

Third generation IUD

These devices act by releasing a hormone. The currently used devices are Progestasert. It is a T-shaped device filled with progesterone. It acts by releasing 65 micrograms of hormone daily in the uterus.

3. **Hormonal Contraceptives:** Hormonal contraceptives are the most effective spacing methods of contraception. These can be administrated orally by ingestion or as an implant. Combined oral contraceptives contain two hormones similar to the natural (COC) hormones in a woman's body an estrogen and a progestin. These contraceptives contain a combination of both estrogen and progesterone or progesterone only. Also called combined pills, COC's, OC's, the pill and birth control pills.

   Mechanism

   - Stop ovulation (release of eggs from ovaries).
   - Also thicken cervical mucus, making it difficult for sperm to pass through.
   - They do not work by disrupting existing pregnancy

   Classification of hormonal contraceptives

   Oral pills:

   - Combined pill
   - Progesterone only pill
   - Post coital pill
   - Once in a month pill
   - Male pill

   Depot formulations

   - Injectable
   - Sub dermal implants
   - Vaginal rings

Oral Pills

(a) **Combined Oral Contraceptive (COC) pills:** These pills contain 30-35 mcg of a synthetic estrogen and 0.1-1mg of progesterone. One pill daily should be taken orally for 21 days beginning of the fifth day of the menstrual cycle. COC pills are not recommended for women feeding the babies, because COC may affect the quality and quantity of secreted milk. Chronic use of COC pills may cause stroke,

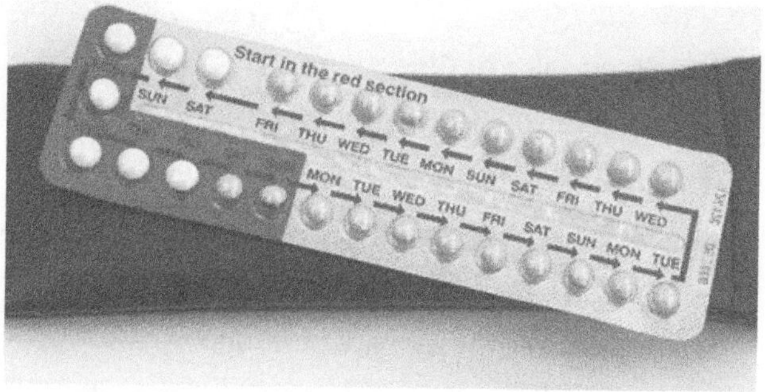

blood clots in deep veins of the legs or heart attack. Women with high blood pressure and are older than 35 years of age and chronic smokers are at high risk to develop the ischemic attacks.

E.g., Mala –N, Mala-D

(b) **Progesterone-only pills:** It contains very small amounts of only one kind of hormone, a progestin. Again, they contain only one-half to one tenth as much progestin as combined oral contraceptives. They do not contain estrogen. These are known as progestin-only pills (POPs), POPs and mini pills. Progestin-only contraceptives are best recommended for breast-feeding women. They do not interfere in milk production. Progestin-only oral contraceptives do not disrupt existing pregnancy.

(c) **Emergency pill:** After an unprotected sex, emergency oral contraception can prevent the pregnancy. Thus they are called as postcoital or 'morning after' contraception pills. Emergency pills mainly stop ovulation (release of egg from ovary) but perhaps also work in other ways. It does not disrupt existing pregnancy. Up to 72 hours after unprotected sex, the woman is asked to take 4 low-dose or 2 "standard-dose" combined oral contraceptives, and then take another equal dose after 12 hours. It contains either a high dose of estrogen or double dose of standard combined pills. Many reports have suggested that Emergency pill have prevented about three-fourths of pregnancies that would otherwise have occurred.

(d) **Once in a month pill:** It contains a long acting estrogen in combination with short acting progesterone.

(e) **Male pill:** It contains gossypol, which is a derivative of cottonseed oil. It acts by decreasing sperm production and sperm count.

Adverse Effects of Oral Contraceptives

Adverse drug effects associated with oral contraceptive pills are

- Myocardial infarction,
- Thromboembolic complications,
- Breast cancer,
- Hyperglycemia,
- Hypertension,
- Jaundice,
- Weight gain,
- Nausea and vomiting.

Advantages

- Ease to use orally
- Almost 100% effective

Disadvantages

- Reduces breast milk
- Side effects and contraindications
- Return to fertility may be failed.

Depot Formulations

(a) Injectable contraceptives: Two drugs are available, they are

- DMPA (Depot –Medroxy Progesterone Acetate)
- NET-EN (Nor-ethiterone Enanthate)

They are progesterone and require administration once in every 3 months.

1. Mechanism: It mainly stops ovulation (release of eggs from ovaries).
2. It thickens the cervical mucus, making it difficult for sperm to pass through.
3. It does not disrupt existing pregnancy

Advantages

- It is very effective; one injection can prevent pregnancy for 3 months.
- It does not interfere with sex and can be used at any stage.
- It has no estrogen side effects. It does not increase the risk of estrogen related complications such as heart attack.

Disadvantages

- These injections may cause weight gain
- Headaches, breast tenderness, moodiness, nausea, and hair loss in some women.
- Does not protect against sexually transmitted diseases including HIV/AIDS.

Contra indications

- Cancer of breast or genital tract
- Unexplained vaginal bleeding

(b) Sub dermal implants: The available drug is Norplant. It contains levonorgestrel. The capsules are placed under the skin of a woman's upper arm. They provide effective contraception for 5 years.

Mechanism: Norplant capsules thicken the cervical mucus making it difficult for sperm to pass through. It stops ovulation (release of eggs from ovaries) in about half of the menstrual cycles after the first year of use.

Disadvantages: Irregularities of menstrual bleeding and surgical procedures are necessary for insertion and removal.

(c) **Vaginal rings:** They contain levonorgestrel which is slowly absorbed through the vaginal mucosa. It bypasses the digestive tract and liver so an effective contraception is felt with small dose.

4. **Post-Conceptional methods**

   Menstrual regulation

   Menstrual induction

5. **Miscellaneous methods**

   (a) ***Behavioral methods:*** Behavioral methods are

   (a) Abstinence (refraining from the sexual intercourse),

   (b) Coitus interruptus (withdrawing the penis from vagina just before the ejaculation)

   (c) Safe period method (avoiding sexual intercourse during day 9-14 of the menstrual cycle. During one of these days the ova may be released)

   (b) ***Natural method:*** They include an increase in basal body temperature during which sexual intercourse should be avoided and the same applies for cervical mucus method.

PERMANENT METHODS

Sterilization

Sterilization can be done for both male and female. The advantages of the sterilization are:

- One time method
- Does not require continued motivation
- Complications are less if done properly
- Most cost effective

Male Sterilization (Vasectomy)

Vasectomy provides permanent contraception for men who decide they do not want children any more. It is a safe, simple and quick surgical procedure and can be done in a clinic or physician's office with proper infection prevention procedures.

During Vasectomy, a piece of vas deferens of about 1cm length is removed after clamping. The ends are ligated and then folded back on and then sutured.

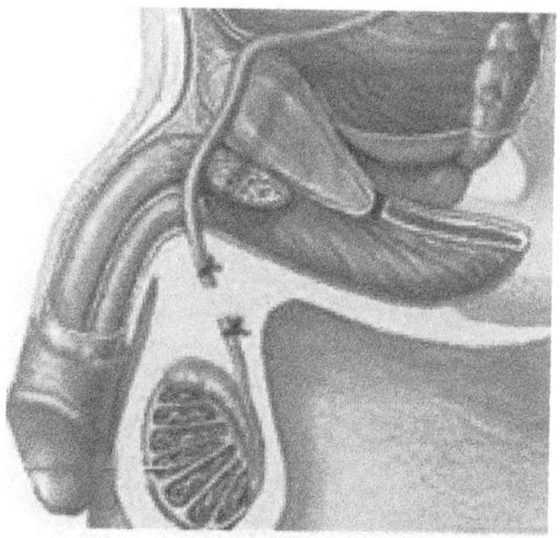

Vasectomy

Complications

- Operative complications like hematoma and infections
- Sperm granuloma accompanied by pain and swelling
- Spontaneous recanalisation
- Psychological disturbance like loss of sexual vigor, impotence, fatigue

Female Sterilization (Tubectomy)

Female sterilization provides permanent contraception for women who do not want children any more. It is a safe and simple surgical procedure and can usually be done with local anesthesia and light sedation. It is done by two procedures:

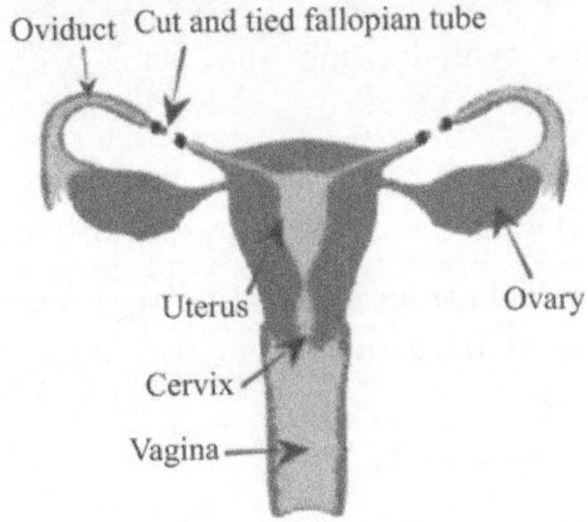

Laparoscopy

It is done through abdominal approach with a specialized instrument called laparoscope. The abdomen is inflated with gas then the instrument is introduced in to abdomen cavity to visualize the fallopian tubes. The tubes are occluded with fallopian rings.

Advantages are short operating time, shorter stay in hospital and a small scar. Rarely complications may develop.

Mini Laparotomy

It is a modification of abdominal Tubectomy. It is a very simple procedure, which requires a very small incision, it is safe, efficient and easy procedure with less complications.

ROLE OF PHARMACIST IN FAMILY PLANNING

Pharmacist serves as a link between public and doctors. Therefore it is likely that pharmacist can come across a number of people with their own beliefs about family planning. The illiterate or less educated people are not aware of the benefits and ease of family planning. Most of them have a psychic fear that sterilization is painful, dangerous and harmful to health. The pharmacist can play a vital role in dispelling these fears.

Pharmacist can promote family planning by:

- Displaying family planning posters in hospitals and drug stores
- Advising people about the importance of family planning, spacing of children etc
- By distributing pamphlet about family planning
- Explaining about oral contraceptives and family planning techniques

India is a country with more than one billion population and second to China. Population explosion affects the country's resources. Thus pharmacist can control this rising population through counseling the people and conducting educational programs that highlight the problems associated with high population. Pharmacist can assist the individuals and couples to know about various family planning measures that are available in the market at affordable prices. Pharmacist can educate the people and convince them about the advantages of having small families.

SUGGESTED READINGS

1. Chez RA.The role of the pharmacist in family planning. A Pennsylvania survey. J Am Pharm Assoc. 1972 Sep; 12(9):464-6.
2. Dr. S B Bhise, Role of pharmacist in the healthcare system. Wednesday, June 11, 2003.
3. Health education and community pharmacy by N. Murugesh : page no: 42-65.
4. Population Reports, Nov, 1989 by Robert E. Lande, Richard Blackburn.
5. Teaching pharmacists about family planning - includes related information.

CHAPTER **16**

ESSENTIAL DRUGS AND RATIONAL DRUG USE

LEARNING OBJECTIVES

- Define essential drugs and rational drug use.
- Know the advantages of having an essential drug list.
- Appreciate method of developing an essential drug list.
- Know the criteria for rational prescribing.
- Understand the role of pharmacist in promoting the rational drug use concept.

ESSENTIAL DRUGS

World Health Organisation (WHO) defines essential drugs as "those medicines that satisfy the priority health care needs of the population. They are selected with due regard to public health relevance, evidence on efficacy, safety, and comparative cost-effectiveness. Essential medicines are expected to be available within the health systems at all times in adequate amounts in appropriate dosage forms, with assured quality and adequate information, and at an economical price that an individual and the community can afford. Essential medicines concept is expected to be flexible and adaptable to many different situations and selection of the essential medicines is the responsibility of the country.

Each country is encouraged to prepare their own essential drugs list considering their local requirements. Presently more than 150 countries have published their own official essential medicines list. The WHO list contains a core list and a complementary list. The core list presents a list of medicines in minimum number that are required for a basic health care system that are most efficacious, safe and cost-effective for priority conditions. The complementary list presents essential medicines for priority diseases, for which specialized diagnostic or monitoring facilities are needed. In case of doubt, medicines may also be listed as complementary on the basis of consistent higher costs or less attractive cost-effectiveness in a variety of settings. The compilation of an essential medicines list helps health authorities to optimize the pharmaceutical resources.

Objectives of an essential drugs list

- Essential Drug List (EDL) forms the basis for national drugs policy.
- Key stakeholders makes health care spending decisions based on essential drugs list.
- EDL serves as a good tool for primary health care practitioners to practice rational drug therapy.
- Helps as a budgetary safety valve for expensive and limited supply of medicines.
- Regular updating of the essential drug list ensures the evidence based medicine practices and current price changes.

The first list of Essential Medicines by WHO was prepared in 1977 and later it was revised once in every two years. The current version i.e., the 18th edition was published in 2013. The 4th edition of WHO Model List of Essential Medicines for Children was also published in 2013.

Criteria for the Selection of Essential Medicines

The selection of essential medicines depends upon various factors such as

- Relevance of the medicine in improving public health.
- Efficacy, safety and cost comparison with other existing similar molecules.
- Requirement of special diagnostic and treatment facilities.
- Pharmacokinetic properties of the molecule.

Most essential molecules should be used as single agents. Fixed dose combinations may be encouraged only when there is an evidence of benefit with combination therapy.

RATIONAL DRUG THERAPY

Throughout the world, ineffective, inappropriate and expensive medicines are often a challenge in various health care settings. This is more often observed in developing countries. Quality use of medicines in the healthcare system is more important not only for economic reasons but also for policy makers and administrators. Appropriate and safe use of medicines is an important element in achieving the quality health care for patients.

Definition

World Health Organisation defines Rational use of drugs as that patient receives medications appropriate to his/her clinical needs, in doses that meet the individual requirements for an adequate period of time, and at an economical price to the individual and overall to the community.

As per the above definition, rational prescribing should meet the following criteria.

Appropriate indication: The decision to prescribe drug(s) should be entirely based on medical rationale and that the drug therapy is an effective and safe treatment.

Appropriate drug: The selection of drugs is based on efficacy, safety, suitability and cost considerations.

Appropriate patient: No contraindications exist and the likelihood of adverse reactions is minimal, and the drug is acceptable to the patient.

Appropriate information: Patients should be provided with relevant, accurate, important and clear information regarding his or her condition and the medications that are prescribed.

Appropriate monitoring: The anticipated and unexpected effects of medications should be appropriately monitored.

Factors affecting Rational Drug Use

In India, various factors such as patients, prescribers, workplace, drug supply system, chemists, drug regulation and industry influence the drug use.

Following are the reasons in each group contributing to irrational use of drugs

Patients: Drug misinformation, misleading beliefs, patient demands/expectations.

Prescribers: Lack of education and training, inappropriate role models, patient pressures, lack of evidence based drug information, company incentives, limited experience, misleading beliefs about drug efficacy, competition.

Workplace: Heavy patient load, pressure to prescribe, lack of adequate lab capacity, insufficient staffing.

Drug Supply System: Unreliable suppliers drug shortages, limited budgets necessitating fixed choices, expired drug supplied.

Chemists Shops: Patient pressures, profit motives, competition.

Drug Regulation: Availability of non essential drugs, inefficient audit system, inadequate legal implementation, and no-formal procedures.

Industry: Promotional activities, misleading claims, incentives.

Impact of Irrational Drug Use

Irrational drug use can have various consequences on patients, public, health care system and even the economy. They are

- Increased morbidity and mortality leading to decreased quality of life.
- Waste of resources, which can lead to reduced availability of other vital drugs and increased costs.
- Unwanted adverse drug reactions and drug resistance.

Some Irrational Fixed Dose Combinations Available in the Indian Market

Sr. No.	Combinations	Irrationality
1.	Norfloxacin+Metronidazole; Norfloxacin+Tindazole; Norfloxacin+Tindazole+Loperamide; Norfloxacin+Tinidazole+Dicycloamine; Norfloxacin+Ornidazole; Ciprofloxacin+Tinidazole; ofloxacin+Tinidazole; Ofloxacin+Metronidazole; Ofloxacin+Ornidazole; Gatifolxacin+Ornidazole.	Though claimed to be broad spectrum, combining (antiameobic) with fluroquinolone (antibacterial) is irrational because patient suffers only from one type of diarrhea. Using this combination adds to cost, adverse effects and may encourage resistance.
2.	Nimesulide+Diclofenac; Nimesulide+Dicycloamine+Simethicone; Nimesulide+Paracetamol; Nimesulide + Cetrizine + Pseudophedrine; Nimesulide + Paracetamol + Tizanidine.	Nimesulide is a controversial drug, has been banned in many countries. It is a sorry state of affairs that its combinations are readily available over the counter. Combining two NSAIDs may increase the side effects of both the NSAIDs. There is little documentary evidence that a preparation containing more than one analgesic is more effective than a single ingredient preparation.
3.	Amoxycillin+ Cloxacillin.	Amoxycillin is inactive against staphylococcus as most strains produce β lactamase and cloxacillin is not so active against streptococci. For any given infection, one of the components is useless but adds to cost and adverse effect. Since amount of each drug is halved, efficacy is reduced and chances of selecting strains are increased.
4.	Domperidine+ Rabeprazole; Domperidone + Esomeprazole.	Increased incidence of rhabdomyolysis.
5.	Simvastatin + Nicotinic acid; Atrovastatin + Nicotinic acid	Probability of myopathy is increased.
6.	Enalpril+ Losartan.	Combining two drugs affecting the same pathway is irrational; it doesn't add to efficacy.
7.	Diazepam+Dried aluminum hydroxide gel Diazepam+ Magaldrate Diazepam+ Dried aluminінum hydroxide gel + magnesium trisilicate+ Dimethylpolysiloxane.	Antacids raise the gastric pH and reduce the absorption of benzodiazepines.

Table Contd...

Sr. No.	Combinations	Irrationality
8.	Cetrizine + Phenylpropanolamine + Dextromethorphan; Cetrizine + Phenylpropanolamine +Paracetamol; Levocetrizine+ Paracetamol+ Phenylpropanolamine.	Phenylpropanolamine is banned drug; yet it's a part of many cold remedies. Besides its potential to cause stroke (more so in hypertensives), it can aggravate diabetes, glaucoma and prostate enlargement.
9.	Cisapride+ Omeprazole; Mosapride+ Pantoprazole.	In patients with gastro esophageal reflux disease, the use of this combination has shown no benefit due to addition of prokinetic agents.

Strategies to Promote Rational Drug Use

Rational use of drugs is an important national issue. The objective of rational drug use is promotion of safe, effective and economical use of medicines resulting in improved health related quality of life (HRQoL) in patients. To achieve this, following strategies may be practiced to improve rational drug therapy

- Most advertisements in many of the medical journals published from India fail to mention important details pertaining to correct usage of drug combinations. Thus there should be a screen on advertisements giving false information to the prescribers.
- Practice of evidence based medicines should be encouraged through continuing professional development programs for practitioners to update their knowledge and skills towards rational drug therapy.
- All hospitals should constitute drugs and therapeutics review committee to rationalize prescribing.
- There should be special lectures on rational drug therapy to the medical students.
- Pharmacovigilance system should be created in every hospital and all health care professionals should be encouraged for monitoring and reporting of adverse drug reactions.
- Every hospital should appoint a clinical pharmacist for promoting the rational drug therapy practice in the hospital.

Role of Pharmacist in Rational Drug Use

Pharmacists can play an important role in rational drug use by providing unbiased drug information to the clinicians, and information on safe use of medicines to the general public.

CONCLUSION

The effective interventions for improving rational use of drugs can be expected from all the members of the health care delivery team. Policy makers should take appropriate decisions to strengthen the medical and all allied paramedical professions to reduce the drug related morbidity and mortality. Government should make appropriate allocation of the resources for better availability of necessary essential and effective drugs. Monitoring of drug resistance and adverse drug reactions will prevent the drug related problems. Promoting rational use of drugs will finally result in improved quality, increased accessibility and better quality of life for the community.

KEY POINTS

1. Essential medicines are those medicines which covers the management of majority clinical conditions.
2. Rational drugs use is the concept of prescribing right medicine in right clinical condition in right dose and dosage form and economical to the patient.
3. Initiation of clinical pharmacy services and practice of evidence based medicine by the doctors make the Rational Drug Use program successful.

SUGGESTED READINGS

1. Essential drugs in Brief. http://www.who.int/medicines/publications September 2001. Issue.No.5.
2. Essential Medicines. http://www.who.int/.
3. The Pursuit of Responsible Use of Medicines: Sharing and Learning from Country Experiences. http://www.who.int/medicines/areas/rational_use/en.

CHAPTER **17**

PHARMACOVIGILANCE IN COMMUNITY PHARMACIES

LEARNING OBJECTIVES

- Define adverse drug reactions.
- Know the classification and predisposing factors for adverse drug reactions.
- Understand pharmacovigilance methods.
- Appreciate the role of community pharmacist in Pharmacovigilance.

INTRODUCTION

Medicines are used to treat diseases. However besides producing the desired therapeutic activity, sometimes medicines may produce unintended, unwanted and unpleasant effects in some people in normal therapeutic doses. Such unwanted drug effects are called as adverse drug reactions. World Health Organization (WHO) defines Adverse Drug Reaction (ADR) as "any reaction which is noxious, unintended, and occurs at doses normally used in man for prophylaxis, diagnosis, or therapy of the disease, or for the modification of physiological function".

Classification of ADRs

Adverse drug reactions are basically classified into Type A and Type B reactions based on the dose and severity.

Type A (Augmented): Type A adverse drug reactions are commonly called as dose dependent and are related to the pharmacological actions of the drug. Type A reactions are usually reversible when the responsible drug is stopped or the dose of the drug is reduced. In Type A reactions, the mortality rate is less but the incidence rate is high.

E.g., Hypoglycemia caused by oral hypoglycemic agents (decrease in blood glucose level than the normal), bradycardia caused by Beta blockers (Atenolol, Metaprolol) Hypotension (decreased blood pressure) induced with alpha blockers such as Prazosin, Terazosin.

Type B: Type B reactions are called as bizarre reactions and also called as "drug allergy" reactions. These reactions are non dose dependent. They are idiosyncratic and cannot be predicted from the pharmacological actions of the drug. The mortality rate is often high with type B reactions.

E.g., Penicillin induced anaphylactic reaction.

Rash, itching or skin eruptions due to quinoline type of antibiotics.

Potential Risk Factors for Developing ADRs

It is very difficult to predict which patient may develop an ADR. However the following factors are considered as risk factors for developing ADRs.

- Age
- Gender
- Intercurrent disease{patient with multiple diseases (heart disease with diabetes and kidney failure)}
- Genetic polymorphism
- Inadequate patient knowledge
- Allergy
- Inappropriate dosing
- Multiple drug therapy
- Prolonged therapy
- Pregnancy

Age: Drugs are converted into inactive metabolites by the liver (detoxification) and cleared from the body through kidney. Liver and Kidney functions are poorly developed in neonates and in young children. Similarly, in elderly individuals, liver and kidney functions become weak. So when drugs are given to these patients, drugs may not be converted into inactive form or sufficiently cleared from the body leading to drug accumulation. The drug accumulation results in drug toxicity and produce type A adverse drug reactions.

Examples: Aspirin induced Reye's syndrome in children.

Nephrotoxicity due to NSAIDs, Aminoglycoside antibiotics and

Hepatotoxicity due to antitubercular drugs in elderly patients.

Gender: Many research studies have reported that women are at greater risk to develop ADRs compared to men due to unknown reasons.

Examples: Chloramphenicol induced aplastic anemia is more common in women patients than male patients.

Multiple and intercurrent diseases: Patients with multiple diseases (hypertension with diabetes or hypertension with kidney failure) are at an increased risk for developing ADRs due to multiple drug use for their diseases. When multiple drugs are used, drug interactions may occur. Due to altered kinetics, concentration of a drug may be increased by the other drug leading to drug toxicity. Similarly patients with impaired hepatic or renal function also will be higher risk for developing ADRs.

Example: Patients with decreased renal function treated with aminoglycosides (gentamycin, amikacin) are at an increased risk for developing ADR, due to decreased clearance (removal) of the drug from the body.

Genetic polymorphism: It is evident that ADRs are more common in genetically impaired individuals. Due to genetic abnormalities, the drug handling capacity of the individuals may be altered. So such patients are more prone to develop ADRs.

Example: Patients with Glucose-6-Phosphate-Dehydrogenase (G-5PD) deficiency are at a higher risk for developing hemolysis (destruction of RBC) when they use primaquine.

Race: Ethnic differences also may account for alterations in drug metabolism and clearance resulting in drug toxicity.

Example: Nimesulide induced liver toxicity in Americans.

Scandinavian and Chileans are most susceptible to develop cholestatic jaundice with contraceptive pills.

Glucose-6-Phosphate-Dehydrogenase (G-5PD) deficiency is more prevalent in Africans. So they are more prone to develop hemolytic anemia with Chloroquine since they lack Glucose-6-Phosphate-Dehydrogenase enzyme which is involved in inactivation (oxidizing) of chloroquine.

Inadequate patient knowledge: Poor awareness about medications and their use may also act as a precipitating factor for development of ADRs.

Allergy: Patients with previous history of allergy to particular drugs are also at a greater risk for developing ADRs upon re exposure. So the drugs for which patients were allergic should be avoided in the future.

Inappropriate dosing: Any drug which is used over the therapeutic dose may act as toxic to that individual resulting in an ADR. Since the pharmacokinetics and dynamics of the drugs vary from person to person.

Multiple drug therapy: Patients taking two or more medications or OTC drugs are at risk for development of an ADR. Studies revealed that fifty percent of patients taking five or more drugs simultaneously may experience an adverse reaction.

Example: When a patient uses a pain killer along with an antihypertensive or anti diabetic agent (multiple drug therapy), the patient is more prone to develop gastritis.

Prolonged therapy: Medicines used for long time such as in case of hypertension, diabetes, tuberculosis or joint pains may also pose as risk factor for developing an ADR. Also prolonged use of drugs may sometimes cause liver damage, kidney failure, which in turn leads to drug toxicity.

Example: Hepatitis with anti tubercular drugs.

Pain killer (NSAIDs) induced kidney failure or gastritis.

Pregnancy: During the pregnancy, drug metabolism and elimination may be altered due to the physiological changes. So these changes may act as risk for developing ADRs in pregnant women.

PHARMACOVIGILANCE

Prior to 1980, medical dictionaries had no word called as 'adverse drug reaction'.

In early 60's after the thalidomide disaster {Thousands of babies born with serious congenital Phocomalia (limbless childrens)} voluntary adverse drug reaction notification scheme was established between American Medical Association, the American Pharmaceutical Industry and the Unites States Food and Drug Administration (USFDA). Later in 1978, WHO (World Health Organization) has established an international drug monitoring center (UMC) in Sweden (Uppsala) with an objective to collect the ADR reports from different countries and perform causality analysis of the data collected. As on date 117 countries including India are participating in the program.

Definition of Pharmacovigilance

Pharmacovigilance is defined as "the science and activities relating to the detection, assessment, understanding and prevention of adverse effects or any other possible drug-related problems in humans".

National Pharmacovigilance Program

The Central Drugs Standard Control Organisation (CDSCO), New Delhi has initiated the National Pharmacovigilance Program in July 2010 at All India Institute of Medical Sciences (AIIMS), New Delhi as the National Coordinating Center (NCC). However, to ensure proper implementation of this program more effectively the NCC was shifted to Indian Pharmacopoeia Commission, Ghaziabad in April 2011. The Mission of the Pharmacovigilance program of India (PvPI) is to safeguard the public health by ensuring the benefits of medicines use outweighing the risks

Objectives of Pharmacovigilance Program

- To have a close watch on drugs regarding ADRs.
- To assess the risk and benefit of marketed drugs.
- To collect the data regarding safety and efficacy of drugs.
- To create evidence based information on safety of medicines.
- To create awareness among all health care professionals.
- To promote rational use of medicines

Advantages of Pharmacovigilance

The advantages of Pharmacovigilance program are

- To minimize ADR related admissions to the hospital.
- To minimize the drug related morbidity and mortality.
- To decrease ADR related health care cost.
- To generate data regarding safety and efficacy of drugs in the local population.
- To detect rare ADRs that occurs in 1 in 10000 patients (Penicillin allergy).
- To assess the incidence and prevalence rate of ADRs for a drug in the local population can be generated.

Who are the Partners in Pharmacovigilance?

All health care professionals can play an important role in the Pharmacovigilance Program ensuring medication safety in a joint collaborative work of doctors, nurses, pharmacists, regulatory and the patients. In developed part of the world, pharmacists' role is much appreciated. Although doctors are primarily encouraged to report ADRs, but due to heavy patient load and other busy schedules, low reporting by doctors is observed.

Due to sound therapeutics knowledge, pharmacists are considered as ideal health care professionals to report ADRs. Many international studies have shown that under reporting of ADRs can be over come to some extent by the active participation of community pharmacists in ADR reporting. Many publications have clearly supported the contributions of pharmacists in ADR reporting. These remarks strengthen the pharmacist role in ADR reporting. During the counseling process, pharmacist can identify the ADRs experienced by the patients.

Various Methods to Monitor ADR

Following are the methods used to monitor ADRs.

- Cohort event studies
- Post marketing studies
- Case reports
- Case-control studies
- Spontaneous reporting system

Cohort event studies: It is a method used to generate or test hypothesis about ADRs in defined population of medication users. It has an advantage of providing incidence or event over a defined period of follow-up.

Case reports: In this type of studies, ADR(s) that have occurred in a particular patient (case) during the process of drug use are identified and reported.

Spontaneous reporting system: It is a simplest and easy method of reporting ADRs. Most of the countries have adopted this method as backbone of their National Pharmacovigilance

Program. In spontaneous reporting system, patients are being closely watched for any potential ADRs. Any doubt about an ADR due to a drug is sufficient to report as ADR, irrespective of the nature or type of ADR. Spontaneous reporting system also acts as a source of drug safety related information for health care professionals, patients and the consumer organizations.

Advantages of Spontaneous Reporting System (SRP)

- It allows characterization of ADRs.
- Rare ADRs can be detected.
- Detection of early warning and signals of the occurrence of ADRs helps to provide information about toxicities of the drug following its withdrawal.
- It does not interfere with the prescribing habits of the doctors.
- It is economical and especially useful for the developing countries.

Limitations

- Underreporting is common
- There may be a respondent and information bias
- Poor quality in data submitted regarding an ADR

ADVERSE DRUG REACTION REPORTING BY COMMUNITY PHARMACISTS

International Scenario

In U.K. the committee on safety of medicines (CSM) is operating ADR reporting through the yellow card system since 1964. Under this system doctors, pharmacists and nurses are authorized to report ADR.

In United States, the Food and Drug Administration (USFDSA) has been conducting MEDWATCH program since 1954 to monitor ADRs to the approved drugs. In this program all health care professionals are encouraged including pharmacists to report ADRs.

In Netherlands, Pharmacovigilance activity was started in early 60's. LAREB, (Netherlands Pharmacovigilance Foundation) encourages general practitioners (GPs), specialists and pharmacists to report ADRs. A team of experts will review the reported ADRs. More than 40% of ADR reports received by the LAREB are from the community pharmacists.

In Canada, ADRs to drug products are monitored by Canadian Adverse Drug Reaction Monitoring Program (CADRMP). This program encourages physicians, pharmacists and other health care professionals to report ADRs.

In Australia, ADR reporting is operated through the spontaneous reporting system. The Adverse Drug Reaction Advisory Committee (ADRAC) encourages all health care professionals including pharmacists to report ADRs.

More than 117 countries including, New Zealand, China, Singapore, Malaysia, Norway, Japan, Brazil, Argentina, and France have been adopted ADR reporting system at national level. All these countries are encouraging pharmacists to report ADRs.

National Scenario

In India, National Pharmacovigilance Program encourages physicians, pharmacists and nurses to report ADRs. This is a great opportunity for the pharmacists to prove their professional skill. Community pharmacists are well placed in health care system to monitor and report ADRs. When patients approach pharmacists for refilling their prescription, or drug returns, pharmacists can initiate a dialogue and enquire about any unpleasant effects due to the drugs that the patient is taking. At this point, if pharmacist suspect any unwanted effects with any of drugs, he/she can collect more information and report that unpleasant effect as an ADR to the nearby regional pharmacovigilance center through the ADR reporting notification form.

KEY POINTS

- Medicines are intended to provide benefits but due to various reasons they may produce unwanted unpleasant effects called as Adverse Drug Reactions (ADRs).
- Pharmacovigilance is a scientific approach to detect the ADRs.
- Worldwide pharmacists are encouraged to report ADRs. Community pharmacists are in first point of contact for patients and are better placed to report ADRs.
- Suitable training and motivation are the key elements to make community pharmacists as good reporters.

SUGGESTED READINGS

1. Kees van Grootheest, Olsson. S, Mary Couper and Lolkje de Jong-van den Berg. Pharmacists' role in reporting adverse drug reactions in an international prospective. Pharmacoepidemiology and drug safety (in press), Published online in Wiley Interscience (www.interscience.wiley.com):10.1002/pds.897.
2. Parthasarathi G and Olsson. S. Adverse Drug Reactions. A textbook of Clinical Pharmacy Practice by Parthasarathi G, Karin Nyfort-Hansen, & Nahata MC. Orient Longman 2004; 8: 84-86.
3. Rabbur Reza S.M & Emmerton. L. An introduction to adverse drug reaction reporting systems in different countries. International Journal of Pharmacy Practice 2005; 13: 91-100.
4. Ramesh M, Pandit J & Parthasarathi G. Adverse drug reactions in a south Indian hospital-their severity and cost involved. Pharmacoepidemiology & Drug Safety. Interscience. (www.interscience.wiley.com), DOI:10.1002/pds.871).

CASE STUDIES

CASE STUDY 1

Mr.MDH a 45-year old male patient visits a community pharmacy with prescription. He has been diagnosed as hypertensive for first time. He collects tablet Amlodipin 5 mg (1-0-0) prescribed by a physician. After 2 days he again visited the pharmacy with the complaints of headache, dizziness, and fainting when he gets up or move suddenly.

Questions

1. What might be the reason for MDHs headache, dizziness, and fainting?
2. How to manage the condition?

CASE STUDY 2

Mrs.N.R a 48-year old lady visited a Community Pharmacy and purchases tablet Ibuprofen 400 mg, paracetamol 500 mg for her tooth ache. She returned to the Pharmacy after an hour and complained that is felling anxious and finding difficulty in breathing.

Upon enquiring, she revealed that she is recently diagnosed as asthmatic and prescribed Salbutamol SOS, she is a hypertensive since 3 years and she is on Amlodipine 5 mg O.D.

Questions

1. What might have caused breathlessness in Mrs. N.R?
2. How to manage the condition?
3. What advice may be given to Mrs. N.R?

CHAPTER **18**

RESEARCH IN COMMUNITY PHARMACY PRACTICE

LEARNING OBJECTIVES

- Know about the research areas that can be carried out in community pharmacy practice.
- Understand about the evidence based community pharmacy practice.
- Design community pharmacy based research projects.

INTRODUCTION

Community pharmacy practice has undergone many changes from ancient days to the present. The earlier compounding activity of pharmacists was replaced due to the manufacturing of readymade formulations by the pharmaceutical companies. This change has made the pharmacists to look into the expanded roles in patient care. Community pharmacy practice is defined as "dispensing the prescription and non prescription medicines and providing information about safe use of medicines and monitoring the patients for the desired therapeutic outcomes". The whole process of reviewing the prescriptions, addressing drug related issues, counseling the patient for improved medication adherence and health outcomes is called as pharmaceutical care.

Pharmaceutical care focuses on outcomes oriented pharmacy practice that requires the pharmacist to work in concert with the patient and the patient's other healthcare providers to promote the patient's health, to prevent disease, and to assess, monitor, initiate, and modify medication use to assure that drug therapy regimens are safe and effective. The goal of pharmaceutical care is to optimize the drug therapy, achieve positive clinical outcomes and improve patient's health-related quality of life within a realistic economic expenditure. To assess effectiveness of the pharmaceutical care service, interventional investigations are necessary. The findings of such interventions will guide the practitioners to provide the improvised services. Various research studies were carried out worldwide to assess the pharmacists' knowledge regarding the professional responsibilities, the need for pharmaceutical care and influence of pharmaceutical care on health outcomes and health economics.

RESEARCH IN COMMUNITY PHARMACY PRACTICE

Pharmacies are considered as first point of contact for public for all their health care requirements. Literatures suggest that patients visit 5-8 times more frequently the pharmacist than their physician. Thus pharmacists are having better opportunities to interact with patients, understand their health related requirements and provide suitable solutions to improve their health outcomes. Appropriate research methodologies can be adopted to study the influence of pharmacist provided interventions in disease management. Research in Pharmacy Practice is in low profile compared to any other areas of pharmaceutical research. In recent times, governments started recognizing the influence of pharmaceutical care on health outcomes and funding the pharmacy practice research.

Pharmacy practice research is defined as "research which attempts to inform and understand pharmacy and the way in which it is practiced, in order to support the objectives of pharmacy practice and to ensure that pharmacists' knowledge and skills used to offer best effect in solving the problems of the health service and meeting the health needs of the population". This broad definition helps us to see the pharmacy practice research as something that can happen both in small scale, large-scale and multi-site projects to improve the understanding of local or practice-specific issues. Research methods are the designs that measures the local health needs and evaluate the effectiveness of services in meeting those needs. A good understanding of health needs can act as a driver behind commissioning new services, in terms of justifying both the need, the effectiveness and value of these services.

Pharmacy practice research should be done systematically on realistic issues that can help both pharmacists and the patients. If the practicing pharmacists are involved in pharmacy practice research, the pharmacists will experience the following benefits.

- Strengthen the quality of the services they provide.
- Build the evidence for developing and commissioning new service.
- Improve the care to patients.
- Contribute to the knowledge within health service research.
- Professional and personal gain in the process of research.

RESEARCH IN PHARMACY SETTINGS

As patients are center focused and all pharmacy practitioners are expected to strive to improve the quality of their existing services and try to develop new ones to benefit the patients both in community pharmacy and hospital pharmacy settings. The research is also needed to assess the work force requirement, educational requirements, and practice requirements to meet the health care demands. In majority countries, the evidences pertaining to the pharmaceutical care services and their benefits available are limited and may be as academic publications. In UK, USA and Australia, the governments have formed the commissions to know the practice status and allocated funds for further research. In many developing countries where pharmacy practice is in low profile, sharing the practice evidences through presentations in professional meetings and journal publications will help the researchers from developing countries to design good pharmacy practice projects.

In community pharmacy settings, availability of more number of patients and practitioners is a good advantage to carry out community pharmacy based research projects. Initially the designed projects may be pilot scale in nature to know the health needs of the patients or effectiveness of a service. Based on the findings, large scale projects may be designed covering the large patient population. The findings of such projects may influence wider service development and overall development of the pharmacy profession.

The department of Health, UK in its 2008 pharmacy white paper states that "In order for pharmacy to become an established voice in primary care and to be recognized as a key and essential element in the delivery of clinical services, a sound evidence base that demonstrates how pharmacy delivers effective, high quality and value for money services is needed". Improving the public health with minimum expenditures is the objective of many governments. Rational and safe use of medicines will save unwanted health care expenditures.

Status of Community Pharmacy Practice Research in Developed Countries

Over the years, community pharmacy practice based research studies were increased worldwide to show the evidences of pharmaceutical care practice on economic, clinical and humanistic outcomes (ECHO). In a bibliometric review of published articles in pubmed shows that, several studies were published using prospective/randomized/single group/pretest-post test designs. Among the studies conducted, majority studies focused on the influence of pharmaceutical care services on economic, clinical and health outcomes. Few studies focused on dispensing practices of community pharmacists, influence of workload statistics on patient safety while filling the prescriptions. In studies conducted covering the pharmaceutical care area include patient counseling outcomes on medication adherence behaviour, treatment goals and health related quality of life. Studies were also conducted on improving the drug therapy in elderly, safe and effective use of medicines.

Research Studies on Patient Counseling and its Influence on Health Outcomes

Information to patients on safe use of medicines empowers them to use their medicines effectively and derive the anticipated benefits such as improved health outcomes and health related quality of life. Various research studies have corroborated the positive influence of counseling on health outcomes.

The Fremantle Diabetes Study examined the effect of a 12-month pharmaceutical care (PC) program on vascular risk in type 2 diabetes. In this study patients were randomized to PC or usual care. PC patients had face-to-face goal-directed medication and lifestyle counseling at baseline and at 6 and 12 months plus 6-weekly telephone assessments and provision of other educational material. The main outcome measure was change in HbA(1c). The study concluded that the 12-month PC program in type 2 diabetes reduced glycemia and blood pressure. Pharmacist involvement contributed for a positive improvement in HbA(1c) independent of pharmacotherapeutic changes.

A Dubai based study conducted by Nadia Rashid et. al., to assess the pharmacist mediated counseling influence on diabetes patients. The findings of the study has shown an improved glyceamic control and reduced cardiovascular risk.

While studying the influence of clinical pharmacist provided counseling on diabetes management, Cioffi et. al., have observed a good glycemic control and improved cardiovascular and renal parameters in patients with type 2 diabetes.

Gerber et. al., conducted a study to assess the impact on healthcare utilization and costs of pharmacist consultations provided to patients with diabetes. The study findings suggest that pharmacist consultations provided to the patients with diabetes has decreased total healthcare costs in a health maintenance organization.

Cranor et. al., had assessed the persistence of outcomes for up to 5 years following the initiation of community-based pharmaceutical care services (PCS) for patients with diabetes. A quasi-experimental, longitudinal pre-post cohort study was conducted in twelve community pharmacies in Asheville, N.C. The study had concluded that, diabetic patients who received the pharmaceutical care services shown an improvement in HbA(1c), and decrease in mean total direct medical costs.

Impact of a specially designed patient education program on diabetes-related knowledge and compliance of insulin dependent diabetic patients was investigated by Powell et. al., The program was successful in improving in both knowledge and compliance among the study population.

Odegard et. al., evaluated the effect of a pharmacist intervention on improving diabetes control; secondary endpoints were medication appropriateness and self-reported adherence. Seventy-seven subjects, were randomized to receive the pharmacist intervention (n = 43) or usual care (n = 34) for 6 months, followed by a 6-month usual-care observation period for both groups. The study concluded that pharmacist intervention had made a non significant improvement in diabetes control with fewer physician visits.

Kiel and McCord evaluated the changes in clinical outcomes for patients enrolled in a pharmacist-coordinated diabetes management program. Data collection included baseline and follow-up values for HbA(1c) and lipids as well as frequency of adherence to preventive care, including annual foot and eye examinations and daily aspirin therapy. The study concluded that the pharmacist-coordinated diabetes management program was effective in improving clinical markers for enrolled patients. Significant improvements were observed in HbA(1c) and LDL values as well as in the adherence behavior to preventive care.

Similar studies were also conducted to assess the influence of patient counseling in patients with hypertension. Agnieszka.S et. al., studied the influence of pharmacist provided education to the patients with hypertension observed a significant improvement in knowledge, attitudes and practices in patients who received education and an improved goal blood pressure compared to the patients usually followed in other community pharmacies.

HEALTH RELATED QUALITY OF LIFE (HRQOL)

Concept of health-related quality of life (HRQOL) and its determinants have evolved since the 1980s to encompass those aspects of overall quality of life that can be clearly shown to affect both physical and mental health. On individual level, this includes physical and mental health perceptions and their correlates-including health risks and conditions, functional status, social support, and socioeconomic status. On community level, HRQOL includes resources, conditions, policies, and practices that influence a population's health perceptions and functional status.

Various community pharmacy based research studies were conducted to assess the influence of pharmacist mediated education on health related quality of life in patients suffering from chronic diseases like diabetes, hypertension, asthma and arthritis using various general or disease specific HRQOL questionnaires. E.g., Short Form (SF)-12 and SF-36. SF-36 is a multi-purpose, short-form health survey with only 36 questions. It yields an 8-scale profile of functional health and well-being scores as well as psychometrically-based physical and mental health summary measures and a preference-based health utility index. SF-36, was designed to make improvements to the original instrument. EuroQol (EQ-5D) is used in a substantial number of clinical and population studies. The Quality of Well-Being Scale (QWB) has been used in numerous clinical trials and studies over the years to evaluate medical and surgical therapies in conditions such as chronic obstructive pulmonary disease, HIV, cystic fibrosis, diabetes mellitus, atrial fibrillation, lung transplantation, arthritis, end stage renal disease, cancer, depression, and several other conditions. The Health Utilities Index (HUI) is a family of generic health status and health related quality of life measure

Indian based Research Studies

In order to assess the research publications in the area of Community Pharmacy Practice, a bibliometric review of publications was conducted by SC Basak and D. Sathyanarayana. Their findings suggest that very little research was done in the area of community pharmacy practice. The areas of research publications included patient counseling, medication adherence behaviour, health related quality of life, health screening services and pharmacovigilance.

Few community pharmacy based studies in India have shown the positive influence of patient counseling in improving the medication adherence, therapeutic outcomes and overall quality of life in diabetes and hypertensive patients and inhaler usage behaviour in asthma patients. Role of community pharmacists in pharmacovigilance was also studied. The findings of the study have shown that, community pharmacists can play a vital role in monitoring and reporting the ADRs in ambulatory patients.

Future Needs

In recent times with the introduction of pharmacy practice courses at undergraduate and post graduate level in India, ample opportunities are available for research in community pharmacy practice area. Both short term and long term research projects may be conducted in large number to ascertain the practice evidences.

KEY POINTS

- Systematic interventional investigations help in understanding the clients' needs, and strengthen the quality of services.

- Research helps in building the evidences base for developing and commissioning new services
- Research findings contribute to the knowledge base within health service research

SUGGESTED READINGS

1. Cheng Y, Raisch DW, Borrego ME, Gupchup GV. Economic, clinical, and humanistic outcomes (ECHOs) of pharmaceutical care services for minority patients: a literature review. Res Social Adm Pharm. 2013 May-Jun;9(3):311-29.
2. Hemingway H, Stafford M, Stansfeld S, et al. 1997. Is the SF-36 a valid measure of change in population health? Results from the Whitehall II study. BMJ 315: 1273–9.
3. Jupiter EF, Guyatt GH, Epstein RS, Ferrie PJ et al. Evaluation of impairment of health related quality of life in asthma: development of a questionnaire for use in clinical trials. Thorax. 1992;47:76-83.
4. Puneeth K Singhal, Dennis W Raisch, Gireesh V Gupchup. The Impact of Pharmaceutical Services in Community and Ambulatory Care Settings: Evidence and Recommendations for Future Research. Annals of Pharmacotherapy. 1999; 33(12):1336-1355.
5. Stroke specific quality of life questionnaire. http://www.strokecenter.org/wp-content/uploads /2011/07/Stroke-Specific-Quality-of-Life-Scale.pdf.
6. WHO Health Related quality of life questionnaire. http://www.who.int/mental_ health/media/68.pdf.

CHAPTER **19**

CODE OF ETHICS FOR COMMUNITY PHARMACISTS

LEARNING OBJECTIVES

- Understand the principles that form the fundamental basis of the roles and responsibilities of pharmacists' relation to trade and profession.
- Know the pharmacist's oath

INTRODUCTION

The traditional functions of pharmacist is compounding, dispensing medicines to the patients in a safe and reliable manner in the interest of public health. By the end of nineteenth century, the practice of pharmacy in the United States has emerged as a socially necessary function sanctioned by the society. These sanctions took the form of licensure laws and examination procedures that established bench marks for professional practice. Pharmacists were comfortable in compounding and dispensing the medicines to their patients on physician prescriptions. However introduction of finished pharmaceutical formulations in unit dosage forms by pharmaceutical companies and chain pharmacies have posed big threat to the pharmacists. During 70's clinically oriented pharmacy practice has focused the pharmacists to provide an effective drug therapy to the patients. Introduction of the Doctor of Pharmacy (Pharm D) programs has made the pharmacists to offer clinical pharmacy services. This has given an opportunity for the pharmacist to be part of the evidence based medicine practice along with clinicians. In the process of this, the pharmacist-patient relationships have become much valuable and important. This has mandated pharmacists to incorporate human values in to the practice. Thus pharmacists are expected to inculcate high ethical standards and behave in a decent way to compassionate the patient. The pharmacy associations of every country have prepared their own professional standards for their pharmacists. Following are the code of ethics for Pharmacists given by American Pharmacists Association.

Preamble

Pharmacists are health care professionals who help the patients to use the medications appropriately. This code, prepared and supported by pharmacists is intended to state publicly the principles that form the fundamental basis of the roles and responsibilities of pharmacists. These principles, based on moral obligations and virtues, are established to guide pharmacists in relationships with patients, other health care professionals, and the society.

(i) **A pharmacist respects the covenantal relationship between the patient and pharmacist:** Considering the patient-pharmacist relationship as a covenant means that a pharmacist has moral obligations in response to the gift of trust received from the society. In return for this gift, a pharmacist promises to help individuals to achieve optimum benefit from their medications, to be committed to their welfare, and to maintain their trust.

(ii) **A pharmacist promotes the good of every patient in a caring, compassionate, and confidential manner:** A pharmacist places concern for the well-being of the patient at the center of professional practice. In doing so, a pharmacist considers needs stated by the patient as well as those defined by health science. A pharmacist is dedicated to protect the dignity of the patient. With a caring attitude and a compassionate spirit, a pharmacist focuses on serving the patient in a private and confidential manner.

(iii) **A pharmacist respects the autonomy and dignity of each patient:** A pharmacist promotes the right of self-determination and recognizes individual self-worth by encouraging patients to participate in decisions about their health. A pharmacist communicates with patients in terms that are understandable. In all cases, a pharmacist respects personal and cultural differences among patients.

(iv) **A pharmacist acts with honesty and integrity in professional relationships:** A pharmacist has a duty to tell the truth and to act with conviction of conscience. A pharmacist avoids discriminatory practices, behavior or work conditions that impair professional judgment, and actions that compromise dedication to the best interests of patients.

(v) **A pharmacist maintains professional competence:** A pharmacist has a duty to maintain knowledge and abilities as new medications, devices, and technologies become available and as health information advances.

(vi) **A pharmacist respects the values and abilities of colleagues and other health professionals:** When appropriate, a pharmacist asks for the consultation of colleagues or other health care professionals or refers the patient. A pharmacist acknowledges that colleagues and other health care professionals may differ in the beliefs and values they apply to the care of the patient.

(vii) **A pharmacist serves individual, community, and societal needs:** The primary obligation of a pharmacist is to individual patients. However, the obligations of a pharmacist may at times extend beyond the individual to the community and the society. In these situations, the pharmacist recognizes the responsibilities that accompany these obligations and acts accordingly.

(viii) **A pharmacist seeks justice in the distribution of health resources:** When health resources are allocated, a pharmacist is fair and equitable, balancing the needs of patients and the society.

Following are the professional standards for Indian Pharmacists

Code of ethics are formulated by Pharmacy Council of India which are meant to guide the Pharmacists as to how they should conduct themselves in relation with patrons (employers), general public, co professionals and the patients.

Pharmacy profession is a noble profession as it safeguards the health of the public in concert with medical practitioners. As per the pharmacy act 1948, only qualified and registered Pharmacists are experts to practice pharmacy.

Pharmacy council of India framed the following ethics for Indian Pharmacists in relation to the job, trade, medical profession and the profession.

Pharmacist in Relation to the Job

A Pharmacist should keep the following in relation to the job

1. ***Pharmaceutical services:*** Pharmacy profession (medical shops) should be registered. Emergency medication and common medicines should be supplied to the patients without any delay.
2. ***Conduct of pharmacy:*** Error of accidental contamination in the preparation, dispensing and supply of medicines should be checked in the pharmacy.
3. ***Handling of prescription:*** A Pharmacist should receive a prescription without any comments on it that may cause anxiety to the patient. No part of the prescription should be changed without consent of the prescriber. In case of any change is required, the prescription should be referred back to the prescriber.
4. ***Handling of drugs:*** A prescription should always be dispensed correctly and carefully with standard quality drugs. Drugs that have abusive potential should not be supplied to any one without a valid prescription.
5. ***Apprentice pharmacist:*** Experienced Pharmacist should provide all the facilities and practical training of the trainee pharmacists. Certificate should be issued only to such trainees who have completed all the requirements.

Pharmacist in Relation to Trade

Following are the provisions which the pharmacist should keep in mind while dealing with the trade activities.

(a) ***Price structure:*** The prices charged should be fair keeping with the quality, quantity and labor or skill required.

(b) ***Fare trade practice:*** Fair practice should be adopted by a pharmacist in the trade without any attempt to capture other pharmacist business.

(c) ***Purchase of drugs:*** Pharmacists should buy drugs from genuine and reputed sources.

(d) ***Advertising and display:*** The sale of medicines or medical appliances or display of materials in undignified style on the premises, in the press or elsewhere is prohibited.

Pharmacist in Relation to Medical Profession

(a) ***Limitation of professional activity:*** The professional activity of the medical practitioner as well as the pharmacists should be confined to their own field only. Medical practitioners should not possess drug stores and pharmacist should not diagnose and prescribe. However pharmacists can offer a first aid in the pharmacy in case of an emergency

(b) ***Clandestine arrangements:*** A Pharmacist should not enter into a secret arrangement or contract with a physician by offering him any commission or any advantage

(c) ***Liaison with the public:*** A Pharmacist should always maintain proper link between physician and people. He should advise the physician on pharmaceutical matters and should educate the people regarding the health and hygiene. The Pharmacist should be keeping himself/ herself up to date with pharmaceutical knowledge from various journals and publications. Any information acquired by a pharmacist during his professional activities should not be disclosed to any third party until or unless required to do by law.

Pharmacist in Relation to the Profession

Regarding to the profession, the following code of ethics should be fulfilled

(a) ***Professional vigilance:*** A Pharmacist must abide by the pharmaceutical laws and encourage other fellow pharmacists to follow them

(b) ***Law abiding citizens:*** The Pharmacists should have fair knowledge of the laws of the country pertaining to food, drugs, pharmacies, health and sanitation etc.

(c) ***Relationship with professional organizations:*** A Pharmacist should be involved in professional activities and try to improve the image of the organization.

(d) ***Decorum and propriety:*** A Pharmacist should not indulge in doing anything that goes against the decorum and propriety of pharmacy profession.

PHARMACIST OATH

I swear by the code of ethics of Pharmacy Council of India in religion to the community and shall act as integral part of health care team.

I shall uphold the laws and standards governing my profession.

I shall strive to perfect and enlarge my knowledge to contribute to the advancement for Pharmacy and Public Health.

I shall endeavors to discover and manufacture drugs of quality to the alleviate suffering of humanity.

I shall hold in confidence the knowledge gained about the patients in connection with my professional practice and never divulge unless compelled to do so by the law.

I shall associate with organization having their objectives for betterment of the profession of pharmacy and make contributor to carry out the work of those organizations

While I continue to keep this oath unviolated, May it be granted to me to enjoy life and the practice of pharmacy respected by all, at all times!

Should I trespass to violet this oath, may the reserve be my lot!

SUGGESTED READINGS

1. Charles D hepler and Linda m Strand. Opportunities and responsibilities in pharmaceutical care. American Journal of Pharmaceutical Education. 1989.53;5:15S.
2. Don A Ballington. Pharmacy Practice for technicians. New Age international Publishers. New Delhi.
3. Robert A Buerki and Louis D Vottero. Ethical responsibility in Pharmacy Practice. 2nd edn. 2002. American Institute of the History of the Pharmacy, Wisconsin.

INDEX

D

E

G

H

O

P

Q

R

S

9 789385 433900

Printed at Repro India Ltd.